Get Out of the Way, I'm Dancing

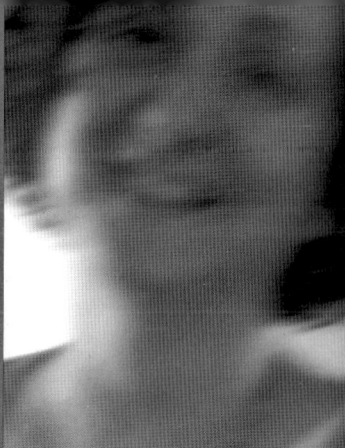

Lauren Singer

Get Out of the Way, I'm Dancing

DOUBLE
STOREY
a juta company

First published 2005
by Double Storey Books,
a division of Juta & Co. Ltd,
Mercury Crescent, Wetton,
Cape Town

ISBN 1-77013-038-1

Cover design by Michiel Botha
Page layout and photographs by Michiel Botha
Project managed by Lindy-Joy Dennis
Printed by CTP, Parow, Cape Town

Contents

Acknowledgements

Many thanks to about the only friend I can be rude and nasty to with impunity. Not that I ever am, of course. And neither is she, indubitably. Barbara Aronson, whose advice and reading of my book in its production phases were invaluable. Thank you, my treasured friend.

My mother and father are my greatest supporters – solid, secure and always dependable. Thank you with all my love.

My dearest brothers, Moishe and Raphy, and dearest sisters-in-law, Deeni and Elana, with all my love.

Chaya Laya, Levi, Dovi, Yudi, Yossi, Chani, Bracha, and Tamar, Natali, Shir, Danielle, Noa, David Moshe – my wonderful nieces and nephews. My links to eternity. You each mean more to me than I can ever express. May Hashem grant each of you a life long lived, full of blessings and challenges which will strengthen you and bring you joy.

Rabbi Avraham J.Twerski who gives me daily strength through his writings in *Growing Each Day*, traces of which are seen throughout the book.

Rabbi Matthew Liebenberg and his wife, Lee, who give me constant encouragement and support.

Rabbi Dr. Ivan Lerner who first introduced me to the concept of **tikkun**.

My nurse, Rukeya Mohammed, and Susan DeVee, my friend and support at home – thank you.

Wayne Gates who, through the years, has seen me grow and fought with me the Battle of the Incorrigible Hair. Thank you for your advice and the final blank pages are thanks to you.

Thank you Dorianne Wiel ('Dr. D') for your wonderful words in your foreword.

Thanks to Bridget Impey, Lindy-Joy Dennis and Michiel Botha from **Double Storey** who took my book and breathed in life and excitement.

Living my life has filled me with an immense sense of gratitude. I would love to acknowledge each of my friends who have given me the joy and privilege of sharing a part of themselves with me. And so I do.

Dedication

To Kathy Robins, Suzanne Ackerman-Berman, Mark Jennings – friends who came at the right time and the right place and continue to make possible a life lived with purpose and dignity.

In memorium

In memory of my dearest aunt, Bubbles Gelfand, who loved books and encouraged me to continue writing in my darkest days. I love and miss you, Aunty Bub.

Foreword

I have never met Lauren Singer face to face, however the conversations experienced with her have been witnessed by thousands. She is a regular caller to my radio show on Talk Radio 702 and 567 Cape Talk. Her comments touch people who refer to her courage, wisdom and above all are moved to look at their own lives.

All of man's magnificent accomplishments seem to pale in comparison with the ability of individuals to transcend the personal crises that they encounter.

With disarming honesty and the ability to confront her illness head on, Lauren offers a real account of an ongoing personal journey from adversity to insight and beyond.

What Lauren Singer has achieved through triumph over ongoing pain and suffering is genuinely inspiring. When shoved against the wall of life, Lauren discovered the incredible – resources of strength, courage, coping and, indeed, thriving that might never have manifested. We are able to benefit from her wisdom derived from intense personal experience. She reminds us that the real life's journey is not upward, but inward.

No one can make you into a survivor and thriver. Only you can do that, but the lessons learnt by Lauren through her journey and shared with us may serve to stimulate thought, engender courage and point us in the right direction. These lessons include an unquestioned sense of priority – a recognition of what is and isn't truly important and assists with appropriate and considered responses.

Too often 'think positively' results in the denial and suppression of real fear, anger and grief associated with personal trauma – with immeasurable negative results. Awareness is always the first step to change. Lauren is deeply connected and in touch with her feelings. She understands what generates them and why and demonstrates the importance of acknowledgement, acceptance and dealing with the truth of despair. Thus she is able to attain self-mastery and move on.

You will be reminded of the meaning and depth of realistic optimism – knowing what is – but still seeing joy and light that is not consumed by illness. This world view enables Lauren to be much more than her multiple sclerosis, to not let suffering go to waste and to become her personal alchemist turning lead into gold in order to improve the present and enhance the future.

There is a wonderful balance between owning and dealing with the problem and trusting and believing in a Greater Power. Lauren discusses the importance of knowledge, taking control and doing everything she can and then surrendering to a larger force which she believes partners her and all of us. In this manner, the finds meaning and spiritual development.

An appreciation of the healing power of support and of the importance of this in her life has enabled Lauren to become a more empathetic and compassionate member of the human race. She reminds us that we are human beings not human doings and never to underestimate the value of simply 'being there.'

Her courageous account of her life, living and dealing with multiple sclerosis is a gift to you that will inspire self-reflection and assist in magical manifestations of resources that you didn't know that you possessed.

Dorianne Wiel – 'Dr. D'
Clinical Psychologist

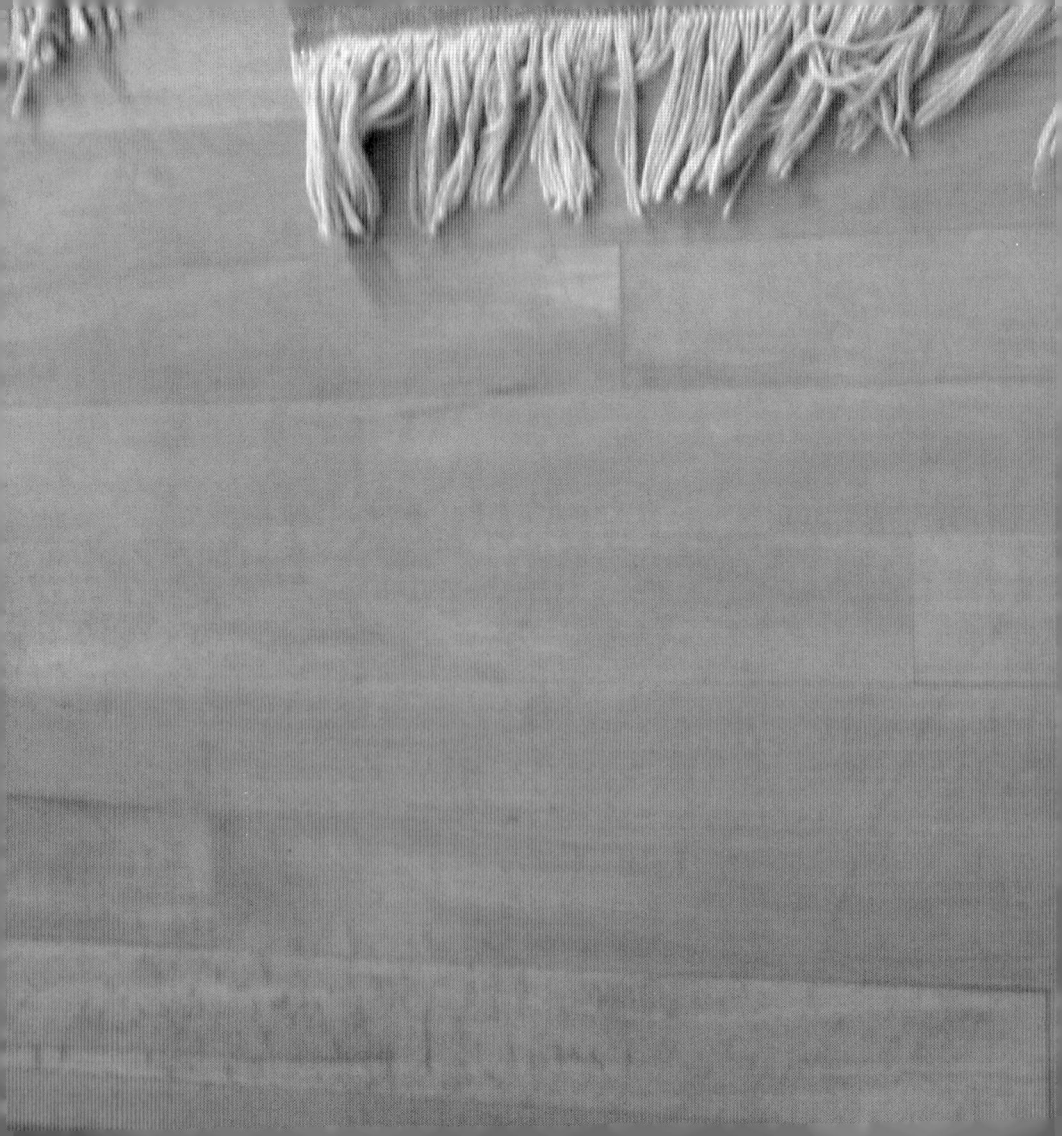

1. Introduction

I feel at the outset that I would like to introduce myself. As I am going on a short journey with you, it is only right that you should know from the beginning a little about your travelling companion. Granted, as you read my book you will come to know me better. If I were to meet you in the street, I would be easily recognisable. I would be the woman with very curly hair, greenish-bluish eyes, and a ready smile. If I were with a friend, undoubtedly I would be chatting and laughing. Maybe we would meet at the supermarket, or at the cinema, or at the mall, or in a bookshop; or in a coffee shop, or at the vet, or at the hairdresser, or at a school.

By the way, I would be the woman on the electric scooter or in the wheelchair.

Your curiosity might be piqued for a moment.
'I wonder why...?'
And if it has been a tough day for me, perhaps I would need your assistance.
'Excuse me, please would you help me. My bag has fallen on the ground, would you pick it up for me? Thanks.'

Then we might start talking. 'Why am I in this scooter? I have an illness. Perhaps you have heard of it? Multiple sclerosis. It is an illness of the central nervous system. You know, the brain and spinal cord? Anyway, the electrical messages don't move easily from my muscles to my brain and vice versa. So, I can't walk very well now.'

It all started when I was 16 years old. I got optic neuritis, an inflammation of the optic nerve. That was the first sign of the pending illness but I was young and the diagnostic tools were not as sophisticated then as now. So although mentioned, I put the idea of multiple sclerosis out of my mind. I matriculated, I started university, went on a detour through two years of medicine (miserable years they were) and eventually found my love of history. After I finished my teacher's diploma, I decided to leave South Africa. The 1980s were claustrophobic and frightening. I was too scared, and perhaps too cynical, to get involved in student politics.

I moved to Israel and I loved the vibrancy, the history and the

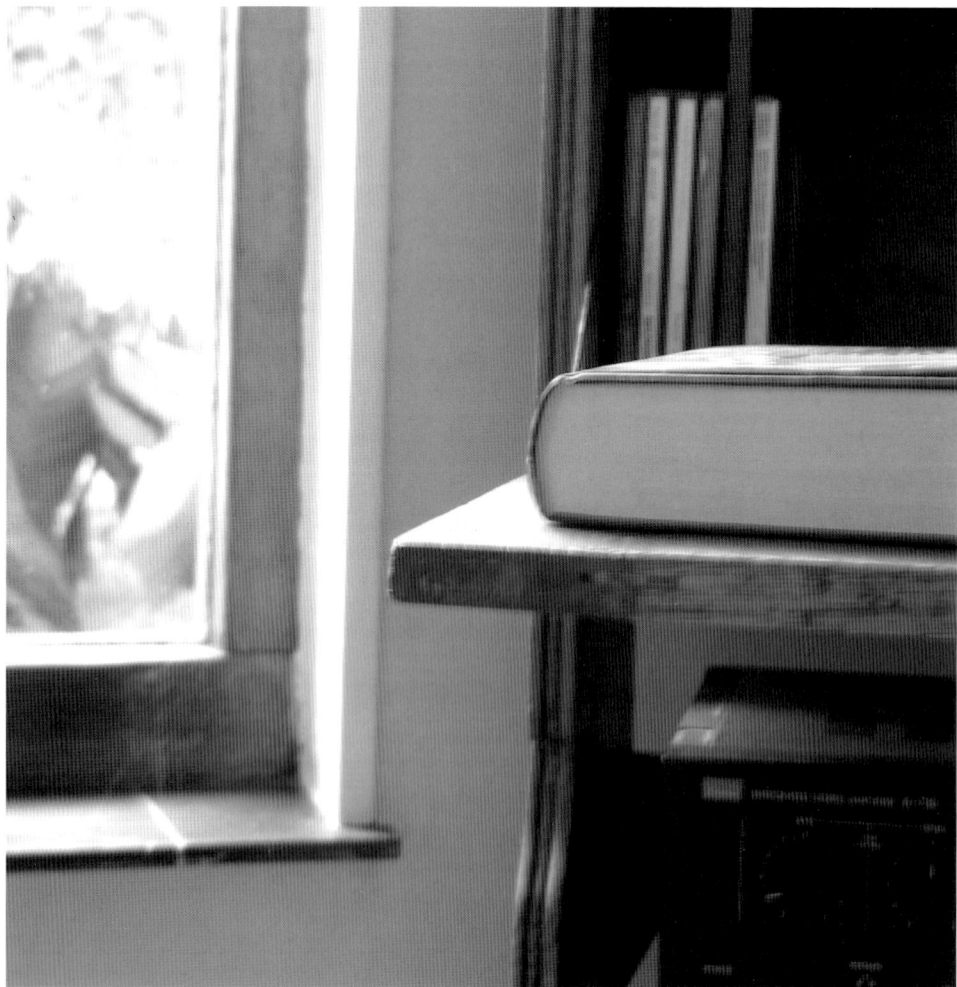

strong sense of belonging. I had been an observant Jew since I was 13 and belonged to a youth group that emphasised both observance of the laws of the Torah (Five Books of Moses and the different rabbinic commentaries) and our love of Israel. What should have been a culmination of a dream turned out to be more difficult. I did not speak Hebrew fluently, which was not an insurmountable hurdle. I went to classes specially designed to assist new immigrants with the language. It was something more than that. I did not have the mental agility, the mental flexibility to deal with the challenges living in any new country demanded. What I did not know was that the mischievous beast, multiple sclerosis, was having its way. Multiple sclerosis does not just affect one's physical agility, it can affect the way the mind tackles everyday obstacles. Nevertheless, I lived, worked and made the best friends ever.

Now I am so proud of what I was able to achieve. I lived in, and I fell in love with, a country made more beautiful by its complexity. I wasn't always so proud of myself – but you will read about that later. After four years, I decided to return to South

Africa. I just knew that I had to return – but for what reason, I had no clue. I decided to study for an Honours degree in history and after that I had no idea what I would do. Three months after my return, I was diagnosed with multiple sclerosis. And with that diagnosis I felt I had again emigrated to another country whose language I could not fathom. I had so much to learn, so much to live.

This book is not about multiple sclerosis. It is perhaps about a condition that we all live with and all tussle with everyday. It is about the human condition. There are no answers in this book – you are as able as I am to find answers and more qualified to look into your own questions than I. Sometimes we all get enmeshed in our own problems. Sometimes our lives are too much with us; our thoughts go round and round in circles. This is a book for those times.

I invite you to come on my journey with me. Maybe you will agree with what I say, maybe you won't. But you will think anew about your own life and maybe you will view it afresh. The book is not complete, however. There are pages at the end of the book that have been left empty. A work of creativity invites your own creativity. As you read the book, add your own thoughts, your own feelings.

Make it yours.

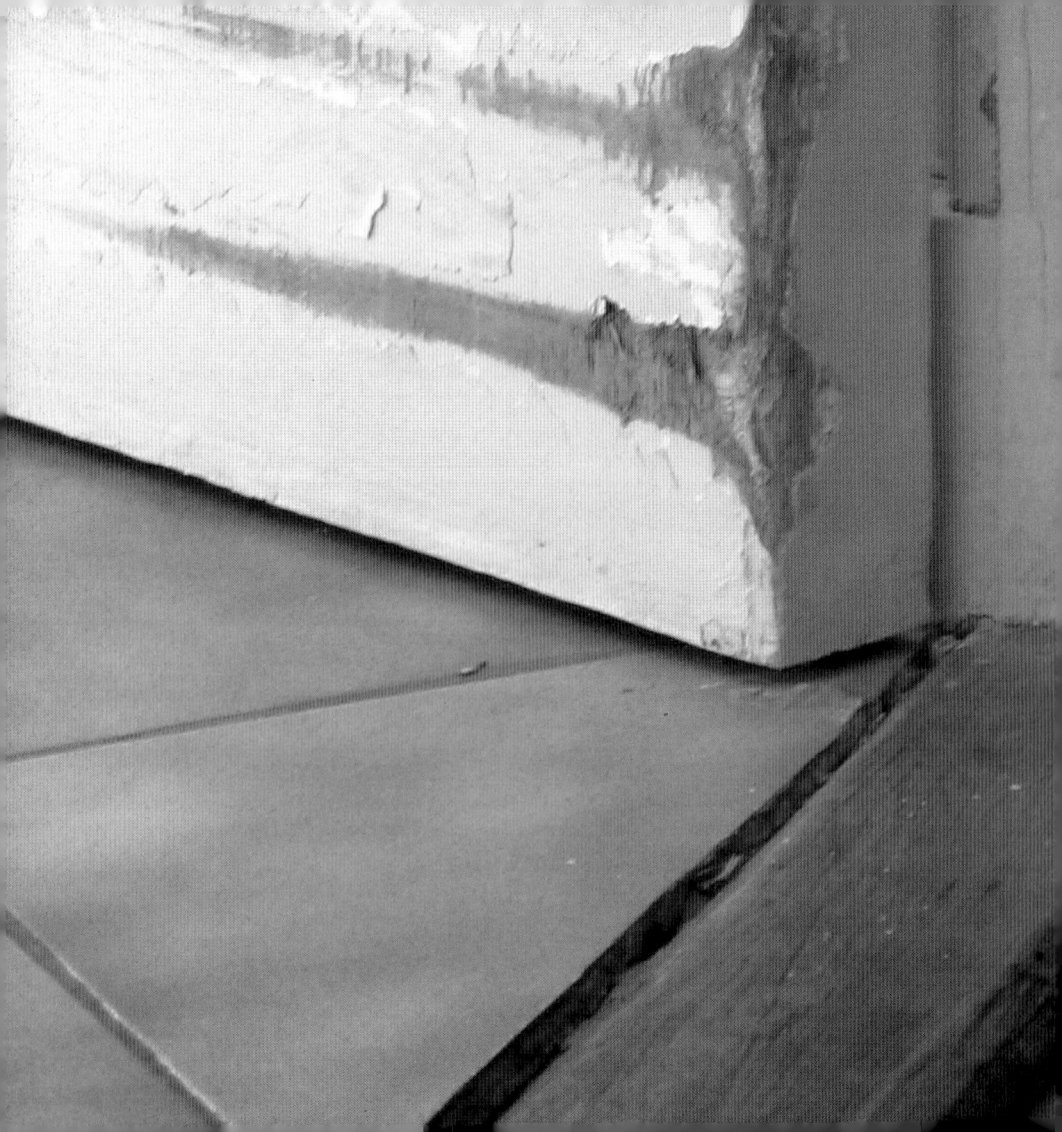

2. Hey, This Wasn't Meant to Happen

I was so proud of myself – I had moved into a flat in Jerusalem, and here I was at my place of work. Six months previously, I had set myself two goals – find a place to live and find a job. And I had succeeded. I stayed in both for three years. I worked as an administrative assistant, a self-styled position – in reality, I was the secretary in a research laboratory in a geriatric and psychiatric hospital. I am by nature a messy and untidy person and I must have frustrated the fastidiously neat and organised scientists. I know that I did.

In addition, I worked with American students who were in Israel for a year. I helped introduce them to their heritage, I taught them the Bible and the wonders of Shabbat. A friend of mine lived in a flat in the Old City of Jerusalem and we would sit on the roof of the building and listen to the muezzins and the church bells and know that just down the road people were praying at the Western Wall. One night I was sitting alone on his roof and I saw a shooting star. I said a prayer thanking God for the wonder.

Walking down a street, or shopping, or just living independently

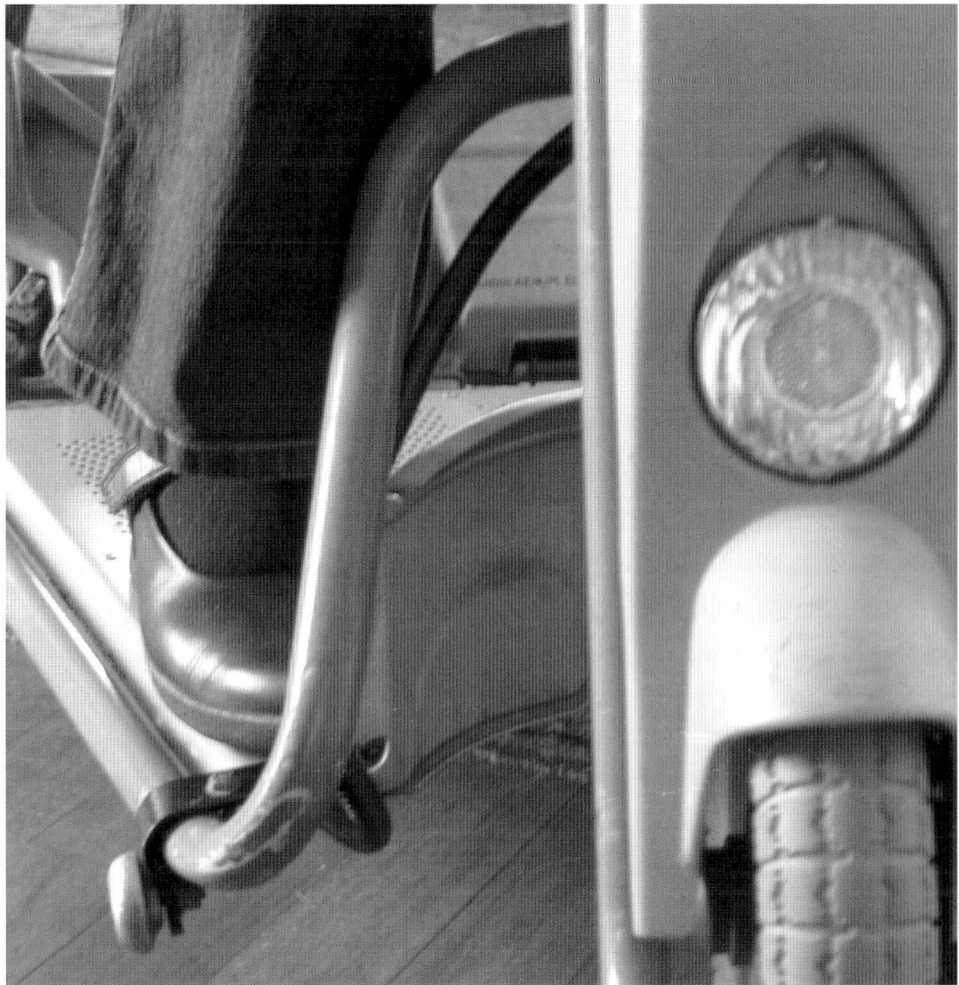

with all the difficulties of life, now seems like paradise. I wonder why I ever left. But I know why. The realities of life had become too difficult for me. I loved Israel but I had became frustrated and angry too. I missed South Africa dreadfully.

I was in Israel for the lead up to the first Gulf War. I had my 'survival kit' – a bottle of mineral water, a few tins of food and a can opener; one room was gas-proofed (sort of) and the bomb shelter (all buildings in Israel have to have such shelters) was readied in case Saddam Hussein sent over scud missiles armed with gas. The impending war did not chase me away – my plans were made long before then. When the scuds did hit Israel, I was back in Cape Town but wept that I was not in Jerusalem with my friends. However, I was back, just in time for the Codesa talks and the build-up to our first elections. Momentous times they were.

Momentous indeed. When I found out, three months after I had arrived back in South Africa, that I had multiple sclerosis, I felt that my life was at an end. My dreams of getting married and having children were shattered. It is not as if I stopped seeing people and meeting new people, but I felt as if I were offering them (men, actually) somebody faulty. Women with multiple sclerosis can and do have children; people with ms do get married. Just not me. At the time I was studying for a further degree in history. I completed the degree, and then what? I was convinced that if anyone knew I had an unpredictable illness such as ms, I would not be employed. Damaged goods, I felt. That's what I am. Therapy did help me tremendously, but what did the trick was my great fortune in meeting the man who would help me change my own perceptions of myself.

I had done a course on the Russian Revolution for my Honours degree. That was a pivotal course for me for a number of reasons: it changed my perspective on the writing of history but, most importantly, it was the impetus that pushed me into a room to listen to a lunchtime lecture given by a visiting Russian professor. Life was offering me an opportunity, but I had not yet come to trust Life again. I did go to the lecture and I met my Professor Apollon Davidson. For the next six weeks, I spent every spare moment with Apollon and his wife, Ludmilla. They went back to

Moscow, subsequently only to return 18 months later to the university to establish the Centre for Russian Studies. I felt prompted to ask him, 'Apollon, do you need a secretary?' He knew I had ms, but he did not hesitate in accepting me. Life was offering me another opportunity. And what an opportunity it was.

I began to gain confidence in myself and in my abilities. My job in Israel had been a preparation of sorts for this job. Truthfully, nothing could have prepared me for the job at hand. I had to help set up the Centre and see that all the bills were paid for the stunning interior decorating. The Centre might have been in the University of Cape Town, but the furnishings went way beyond university decor. The man who was funding the Centre wished it to be beautifully set up. So we had lavish curtains, carpeting and furniture.

Apollon and I went to secondhand bookshops and he slowly and carefully constructed a library of books. I was so proud when I found some books of which he approved. He told me

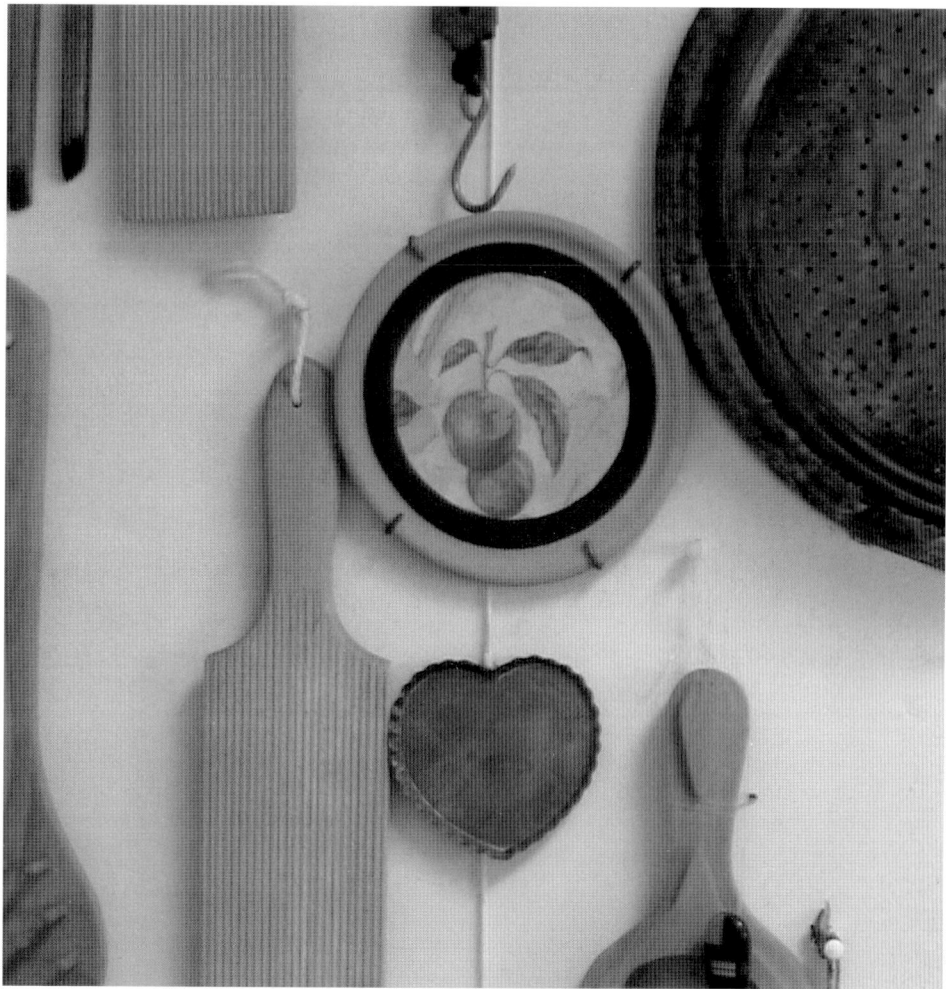

that I had a good eye. I have always felt that books give any room its character, and the rooms of our Centre breathed life and knowledge. I could not believe my good fortune. I felt enveloped by love. Enveloped by my love of history, enveloped by the joy of working with a man I truly admired. I was in an atmosphere of learning and growth. My greatest joy was when anybody came to visit. It did not matter who it was – a visiting Professor from Russia or a visiting student who popped in out of curiosity. Everyone was offered a cup of tea and biscuits.

Professor Apollon Davidson continued his work writing books. He is one of the world's foremost Africanists. His book on Cecil John Rhodes is superlative – it was the first book of Professor Davidson's that I ever read. I played a small role in the publication of two further books. One was on Russia and the Anglo-Boer War. Just to be a small cog in their production was immensely rewarding. My best memories are of us chatting in his office over a cup of tea. There were often occasions to raise a toast and then it would be over a glass of vodka. Stolichnaya – the real Russian stuff. At the end of our first year, we toasted the first student to be given a ticket to Russia for his top marks in the Russian language course Ludmilla had taught at the Centre. Could it get any better?

Professor Davidson was going to present a series of lectures to third-year history students on the topic, Russia in the Second World War.

'Could I be the tutor?' I asked tentatively.

'Brilliant, brilliant,' was Apollon's response.

So I was the tutor: I prepared all the tutorial material; helped set essay and exam questions and helped mark them all. I could not have been happier. I had met fascinating people. Vladimir, or Valodya, was the first Russian vice-consul I ever met. He spoke English with a perfect English accent and I was fascinated. He would come in to the Centre and I would say to him, 'What about a cuppa?' and over a cup of tea we would chat and he would tell me about his life in Russia. At times I felt I was living through a Graham Greene novel. My life had become exotic. But then, after four years, the funding for the Centre dried up.

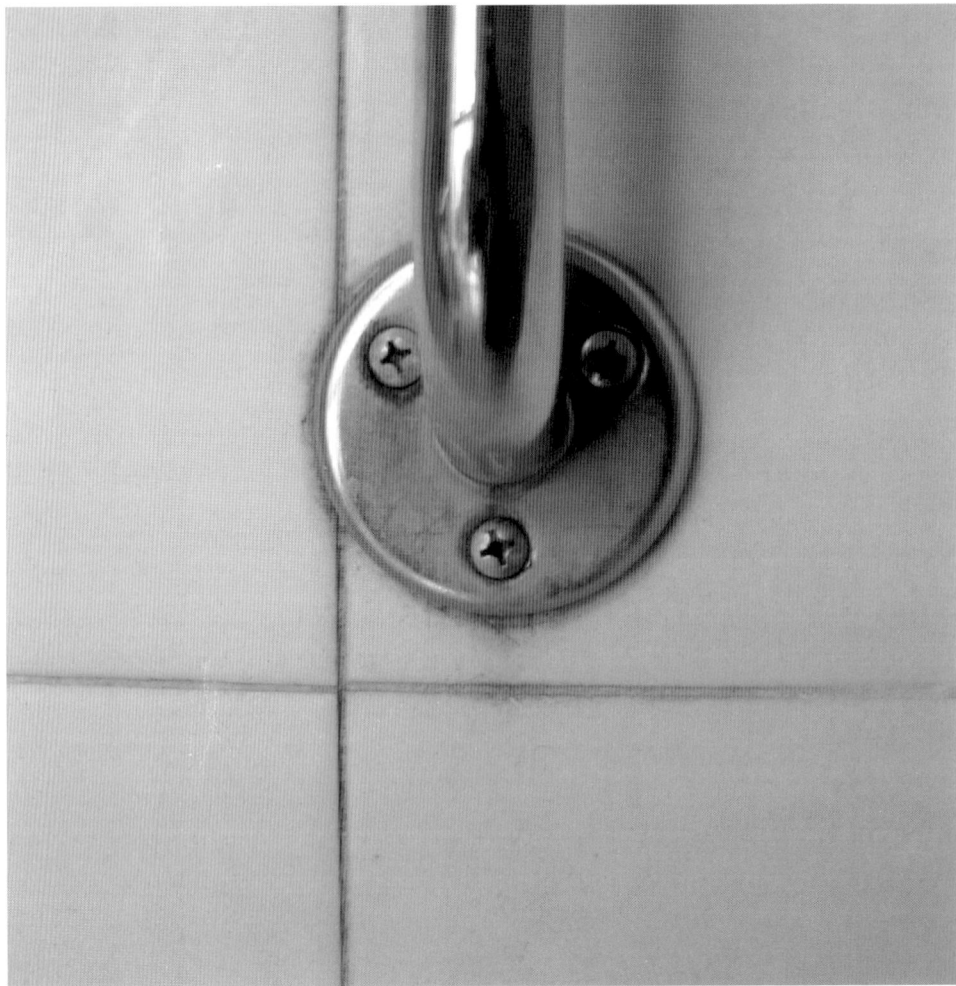

We had to dismantle the library and the Centre, and prepare for the end with dignity. Apollon and Ludmilla went back to Moscow and I had to look forward. I continued to work at the university, but now at the Disability Unit. Apollon had protected me. The Centre had been a gentle eye of the university maelstrom. The multiple sclerosis had begun to affect my ability to work long hours. I had started using an electric scooter at work because I could not walk very well. I first started using Dragon-Dictate (a voice-activated programme that I could use instead of typing) about a year before the Centre closed. I did not work long for the Disability Unit, perhaps six months. I don't think that I ever got used to not working at our Centre. I continued to work to the best of my ability, but that clearly was not good enough. I was advised to take early retirement due to ill health. I was staggered. Distraught. I knew that multiple sclerosis affected the way that I worked, but I had never thought I would be considered incompetent!

I made up my mind: I would get up every morning at my usual time and get dressed as if I were going to work. It was crucial to keep my mind alert and ready to take up any opportunity. One evening I heard an interview about the 'Pink Map' of Cape Town. I was not in the least interested in the map itself, but the concept grabbed me. What about a 'Disability Map' of Cape Town highlighting all the places that were disability friendly in and around Cape Town? I spoke to the man who had produced the map, as well as the Cape Town Tourism Board. Coincidentally, plans were being made regarding the establishment of a company specifically geared to tourists with special needs, including physical disabilities. I linked up with the newly established company, the Enabled Traveller, and was involved in inspecting hotels, restaurants and tourist sites to see whether they were 'disability friendly'. I was then given what had to be the most thrilling assignment: I was to inspect the Elephant Hills Hotel at Victoria Falls, Zimbabwe. How disability friendly was the hotel? So off I went, with my mother in tow to give me physical help, to find out.

The people at the hotel were extremely friendly and helpful. Unfortunately, I could not use the room that they had given me. I needed a separate shower and could not use the bath with a shower head. I could not get into the bath, you see. They took me to see another room, but the carpeting was too thick. I could walk with my walker to assist me, but not if the carpeting tripped me up. There was one more room, they said, which hopefully would suit me. And they led me to the Presidential Suite. The flooring was made of marble; there was a separate shower. I felt totally overwhelmed. 'I feel like Liza Dolittle', I thought to myself remembering *My Fair Lady*.

What a wonderful time we had. We took a helicopter ride over Victoria Falls; we were given a grand tour of the hotel and a ride on the famous golf course. Then came the most exciting adventure of them all: we went on an elephant safari. With help and gentle assistance, I was put on the back of the elephant and off we went. I had never been so close to those patient pachyderms, but to ride on one of them was breathtaking. And do you know they have a fine sense of humour? We had taken a break and were laughing and chatting together. Then one elephant rolled up his trunk and gave a member of our group a not so gentle punch in her stomach, just to show that he, too, was part of the group.

Sadly, the Enabled Traveler project and company had to be dismantled soon after. So, what was going to be my next project? I was contacted by the Disability Unit and given what was going to be a pivotal project in my life. I was commissioned to write a book about multiple sclerosis. I was excited, but I was also rather nervous. It was a book commissioned by a university department, so it had to be academically sound. On the other hand, I was writing about a subject that was part of me. How could I be totally objective? My friend and mentor advised me, 'The more honest you are, the better it will be.' And I wrote a book that was both objective and subjective.

It had not been an easy book to write, but through writing it, I found healing. The book, *A Measure of Time: My Life with MS* was published and has gone into its second printing. With the book in hand I began to speak to groups including groups of schoolchildren about it, and about my journey with the illness. 'From adversity to advantage' was the title of my talk. So I started on my writing career, and also my public speaking career. I met my faithful friend, Fred, when I still worked in the Centre for

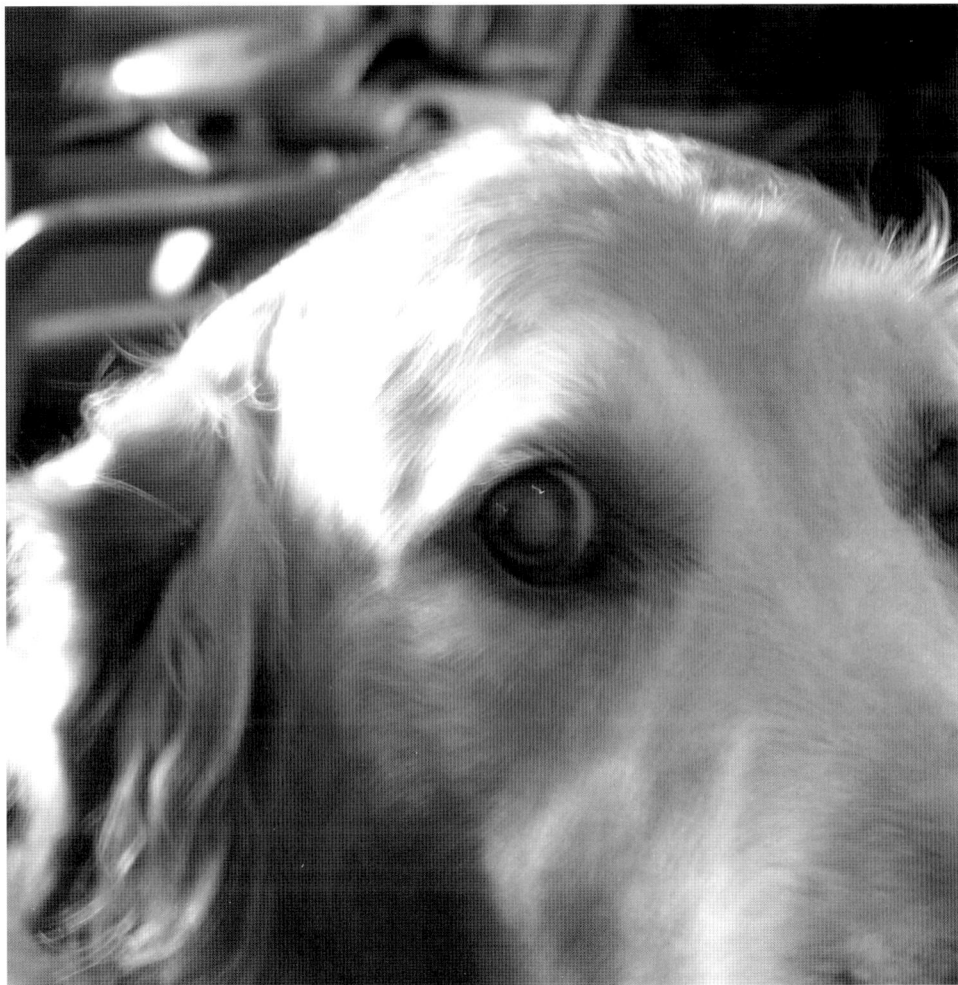

Russian Studies. Fred is a golden retriever and he is the 'author' of my second book, *Fred at Your Service, Ma'am.*

My love of teaching has also found a fascinating and fulfilling outlet. I helped introduce and present a course of lectures on ms to first-year medical students at the University of Cape Town. When I worked in the Disability Unit I met Margi, a lecturer in the Occupational Therapy Department at the University of Cape Town. She asked me to speak to the first year students about multiple sclerosis and about my life living with it. Every year since then, I have spoken to the first-year students on that topic. In the past year, Margi invited me to join her for the entire course she was to present. I was to be the 'disabled expert' who would present real life experience to the course material she would lecture.

It all sounds rather simple doesn't it? Sort of drifting from one thing into another. But it wasn't simple and it wasn't easy. When I was medically boarded from the university, another friend of mine advised me to make multiple sclerosis my career. I was shattered at that time, but what he said lodged in my mind. I have taken an extremely debilitating and frustrating illness and made it serve my purposes. I have worked with it and not against it and I have been able to turn setbacks into advantages. I met the right people at the right time to assist and support me. But none of that could have happened without looking deeply into myself; my preconceptions. Each of us is able to take ourselves, give a little shake, look around and make the most of what we have.

This book is an exploration of the journey I have taken, and am in the process of taking. With each set back I could have said, 'Hey, this wasn't meant to happen.'

But, just perhaps, it was.

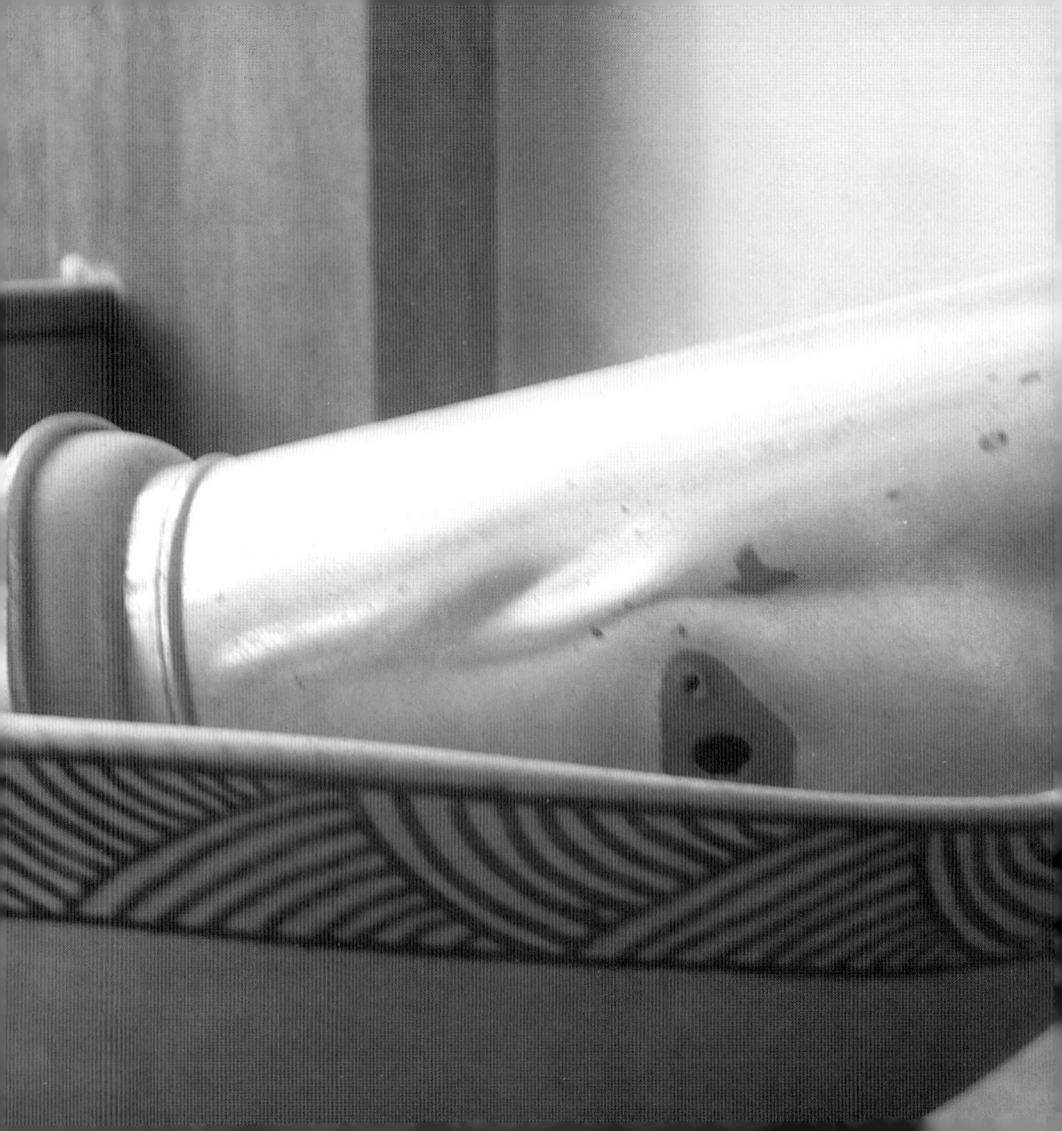

3. Denial Is More Than a River in Egypt

A man is on a hike over hilly terrain. He is exhausted, sits on a rock and takes out his water bottle. Only a little bit of water left, he sighs. He squints up at the sun, shakes his head and slowly gets up. Leaning heavily on his stick he trudges on. He kicks the pebbles on the path and makes a game of it. Laughing, he aims for a tree, misses it and tries again a few paces later. It hits target. Eventually he comes to a crossroads and, sitting on a bench, is an elderly man. Our intrepid hiker doesn't know which path to take.

'Em, would to help me please? I am heading for the nearest village, but I don't know which path to take. Would you advise me?' The elderly man looked up and smiled. 'Certainly. Both paths lead to the village. One is long but short, and the other is short but long. It's up to you.'[1] 'Thanks for nothing,' the hiker mumbled.

Again he squinted at the sun, shook his water bottle and shrugged. 'I will take the shorter route,' he thought to himself.

[1] This story is based on a story from the Talmud *(Eruvin 53b)*

And so he did. He found the path strewn with boulders he had to climb over. Then there was the nettle bush he tripped into. He finished his water just as the sun was setting. He swore softly to himself as he munched his last biscuit.

'Bloody hell,' he yelled as he fell into a hidden pothole in the road. He had twisted his ankle but, swallowing a curse, he stood up and hobbled his way forward.

Eventually he came to the village and was startled to meet the elderly man from the crossroads.

'Hey, how did you get here before me? When did you get here? And why didn't you warn me that the path was filled with obstacles?' The elderly man shook his head. 'I told you that you could go either way. I took the long but short route. It is quicker that way, you know. And how could I warn you of the obstacles? I avoid that route because the obstacles are difficult and the path painful, but the terrain is never the same.'

Read the story carefully again. Which path would you take?

When I first heard the story, it was so clear to me. Obviously I would take the long but short route. I would get to my destination in the quickest possible time. I would not be faced with any dangerous obstacles. It would be foolhardy to go the other way. Only a masochist would voluntarily take the other route. But perhaps the story is not so simple.

Let's go back to the crossroads. The elderly man was in control of the facts. He could make a considered decision. Clearly, he had walked the paths before. So why couldn't he tell the hiker that the one route was dangerous? The key lies in his final statement: **The obstacles are difficult and the path painful, but the terrain is never the same.**

The terrain is never the same and it seems as if it was specially tailored for you. I was 27 when I was first diagnosed with multiple sclerosis. Apparently, my first symptoms started when I was 16. It manifested in the form of optic neuritis

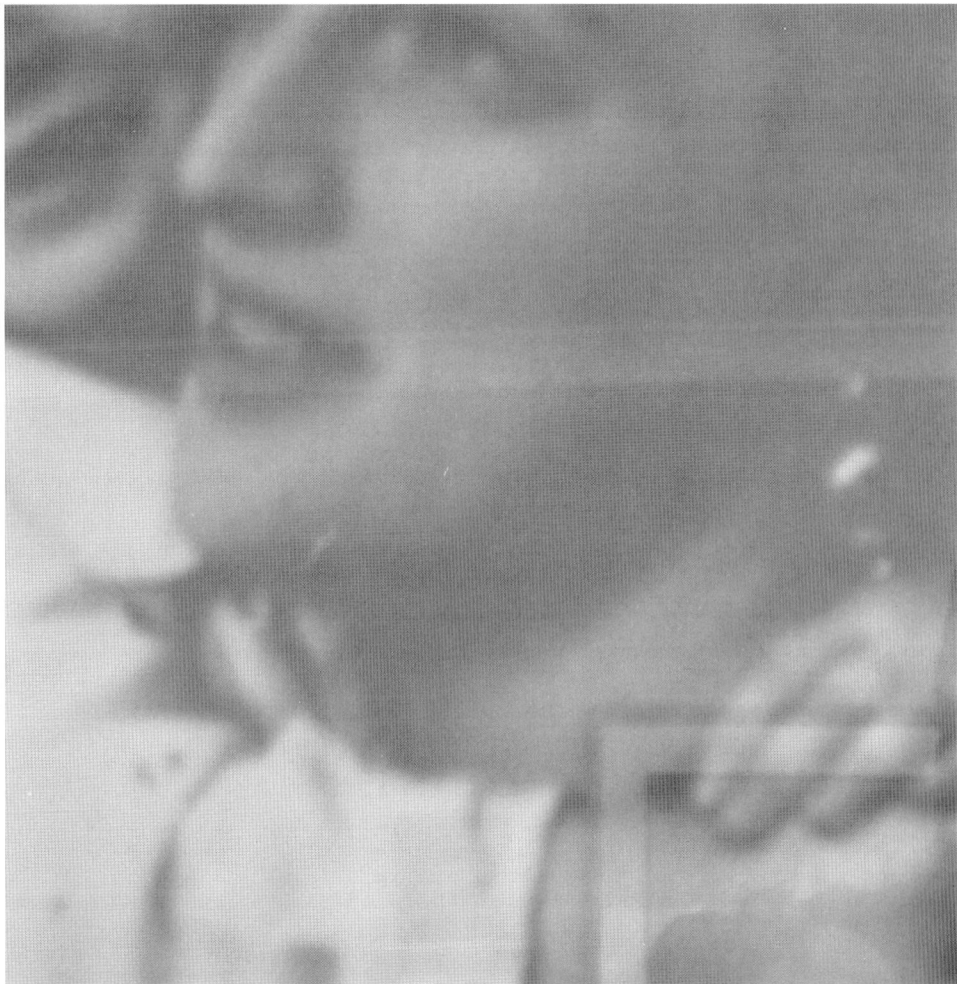

which left my eyesight dimmed in one eye. It cleared up and I continued my life. I have described ms as a 'mischievous beast', perplexing and quixotic. For 11 years, ms went his independent way, chomping a bit of myelin here and there until his presence could not be ignored. I was given a diagnosis that I could not fathom. I could not even pronounce multiple sclerosis and had to keep repeating the words: multiple sclerosis.

So I was at my crossroads. Which was the best path? The short but long was my choice. I decided to fast track my adjustment. Anger, denial and eventually acceptance. Fine, I could do that. Give me three days, I thought. But I had not even touched the surface of my anger and denial was my constant companion. Forget acceptance, I did not even know what it was I had to accept. I carried on my life, finished my degree and remained seething. Denial is such a wonderful companion. It lets you carry on your way and even appears to strengthen you. But eventually it is a hollow companion and the strength it seems to bestow is only an illusion.

When I found out that I had ms, I had to find out the reason why. No one knows the reason why some people get the illness and others don't. There are theories and possible explanations, but, in the end, no one really knows. If I could find the reason why, I reasoned, surely I would be able to get better. This is where denial becomes so insidious. It is the first and most fundamental denial. We fool ourselves into thinking that we have the capacity to be fully in control of our lives.

There are some things we cannot control. It is not a matter of giving up control of our lives, but realising that ultimately we have limited control. Isn't it strange, but in giving up our need to control, we gain control. I started looking for solutions, practical solutions for living. Eating healthily, ensuring I get enough rest and choosing goals that are attainable. I cannot chastise myself for not running the Two Oceans marathon. I can feel pleased and proud of my persistence in walking down the corridor. Some days I can and some days I can't. The trick is to look on both with equal favour.

Knowledge. I needed to know how the ms worked, what was its *modus operandi*? What drugs were available and which would benefit me? What about the expense and the availability? I cannot control the ultimate outcome of my illness. Sure, there are drugs that seem to delay progression of the illness but, as yet, there is no drug that will take it away. But I can seek ways to grapple with my symptoms in the best way possible. All along the way, the boulders and obstacles seem insurmountable. I have learned to approach each obstacle as it comes. I try not to project into the future, but work with my present and with my day.

How can you tell the difference between hope and denial? Of course I hope that a cure for the illness will be found. Hope gives me the strength to continue and to live the best life possible. Hope stops me from giving up. Without hope, life would be untenable. Denial, on the other hand, stops you from looking for solutions. If you cannot see the problem, there is no way you can surmount it. Denial cripples you.

So, have I conquered denial?

No.

In all aspects of my life I try to be honest, to look at myself clearly without self-deception. Once, I had a wonderful friend whom I adored. I learned more from him and was happiest with him than ever before. I just refused to ask questions. I could feel that he had not told me the full truth, that he had kept things from me. His friendship was too valuable to shatter with answers to questions that plagued me. When he died the truth did come out. He had undoubtedly loved me, but he had also lived with a partner all the time he knew me. I had believed he had lived alone. I was broken and had to make peace with my self-deception and denial. Of course I love him still, and am forever grateful for his friendship. Above all I learnt that we all live with denial and facing it and living with the consequences can be very painful.

And what about the basic denial that I spoke of earlier? Have I fully accepted that I cannot control the illness? No.

It is so important to have a sounding board. A dear friend of mine also has multiple sclerosis. When I am feeling low, I tend to blame myself for any difficulties I have with multiple sclerosis. The thoughts always intrude, 'What if I had not given up walking? Perhaps the reason why I am not walking well is because I started using my electric scooter too soon. Maybe it is my fault. Maybe if I had delved deeper I would have found out why I have ms. Perhaps I should try harder to cure myself.' And my friend helps put my life into perspective. We talk and laugh and I can face my life better.

So let's go back to the crossroads. The hiker did arrive at the village. He had to face every challenge head on. He could not turn back. Perhaps there was an easier route, perhaps there was a smoother way. His path was hard and it was painful, but it was his path. He had to grapple with the terrain and nobody who had gone before him could warn him. One problem with the story is that the hiker had to walk alone. We do not have to walk alone. When I was growing up I wanted to be different. Now I rejoice in my sameness. Of course we are all individuals, have our own outlook on life, but there is strength to be gained from the experiences of others. Strength and wisdom.

Attempt to look at your life with honesty
I realise that the primary and first denial is the illusion of control
Knowledge is the key
Seek friends who can help put your life into perspective
Denial is no protection although it may seem that way
Seek the difference between hope and denial

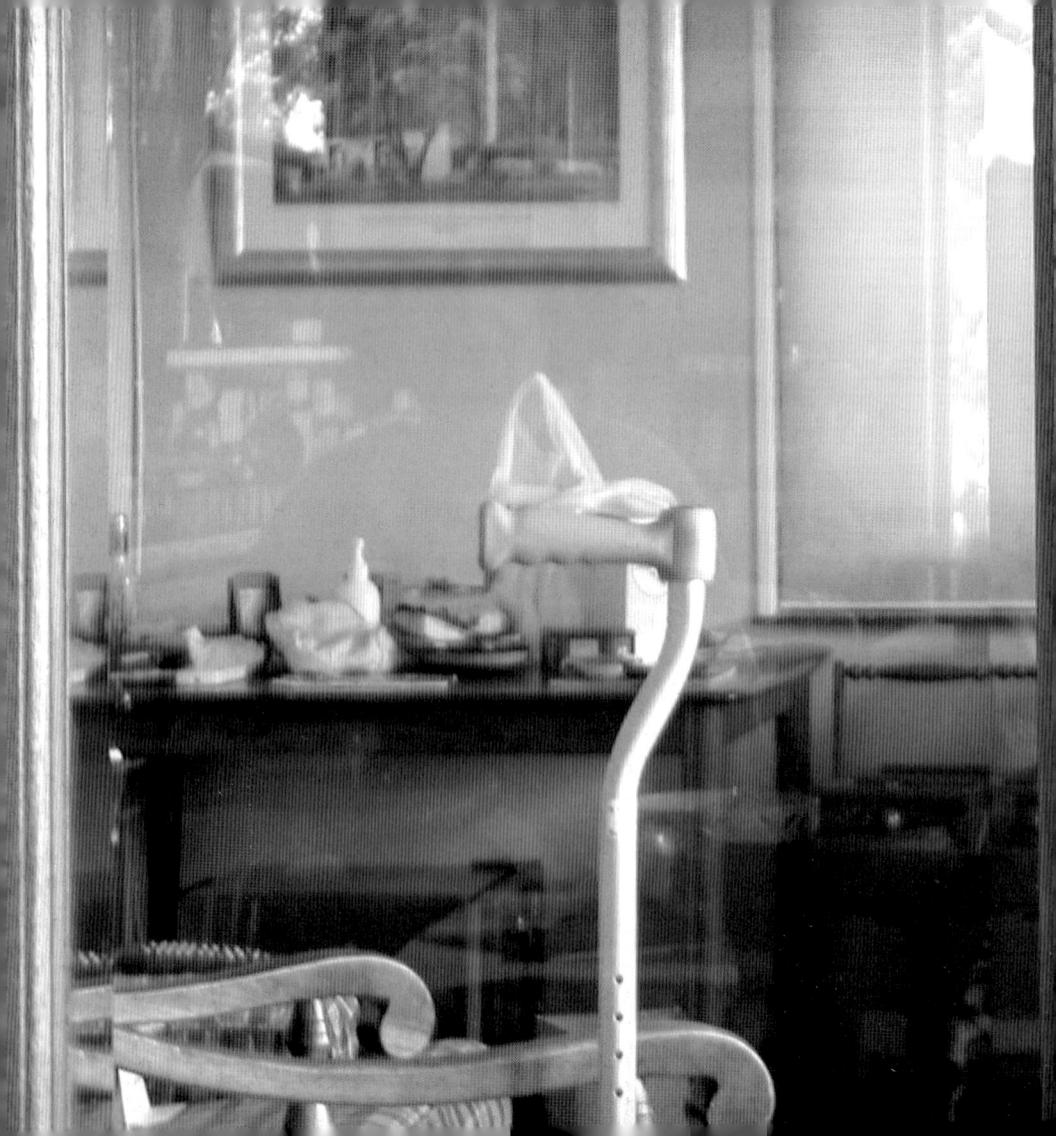

4. So Who Wins the Blame Game, Anyway?

We all play the blame game. When we were children it was easy to point a finger and say, 'It's not my fault. It is Mary's or Jane's or John's.' And as we grow older, the game becomes a little bit more involved.

So I got this horrible illness. I had been back from Israel only a few months and was seething with anger. I did not know where to put my hatred for myself. I felt I had failed. I been unable to make a success of my life overseas, and I had returned home full of self-recrimination. Then I was diagnosed with multiple sclerosis. I was 27 years old and confused. I could not verbalise my frustration but I surely could shout. I would bite my hand and try to hit myself on my head with a spanner or anything heavy, to hurt myself. I was crying inside.

The wise thing, I thought. I will do the wise thing – I will continue my university course (after all that was my reason for returning, wasn't it?). I will immerse myself in my religion. That is responsible, isn't it? And all the time I was crying inside me, trying to make sense of it all.

Then the blame game began in earnest. It all starts with the one question, 'Why?' Why did I get the illness? Or, why did this happen to me?

You see, there was no answer to that question. Well, not yet anyway. There seemed to be answers. Obviously the reason why I got the illness was because there was something faulty in me. There had to be something wrong with me. Spiritually. I had been religious for many years but somehow I had not matched up to G-d's expectations. I had tried my best but obviously that was not good enough.

So then we had it, **I was to blame**.

The problem with blame is that it is so full of shame. So full of finger pointing. So full of anger. I had done nothing tangible. Nothing that I could grapple with and make better. I looked at my personality, and at my many perceived failures and my self-loathing grew. At that time, I was not particularly disabled. I could still drive, my walking wasn't badly affected. Sometimes

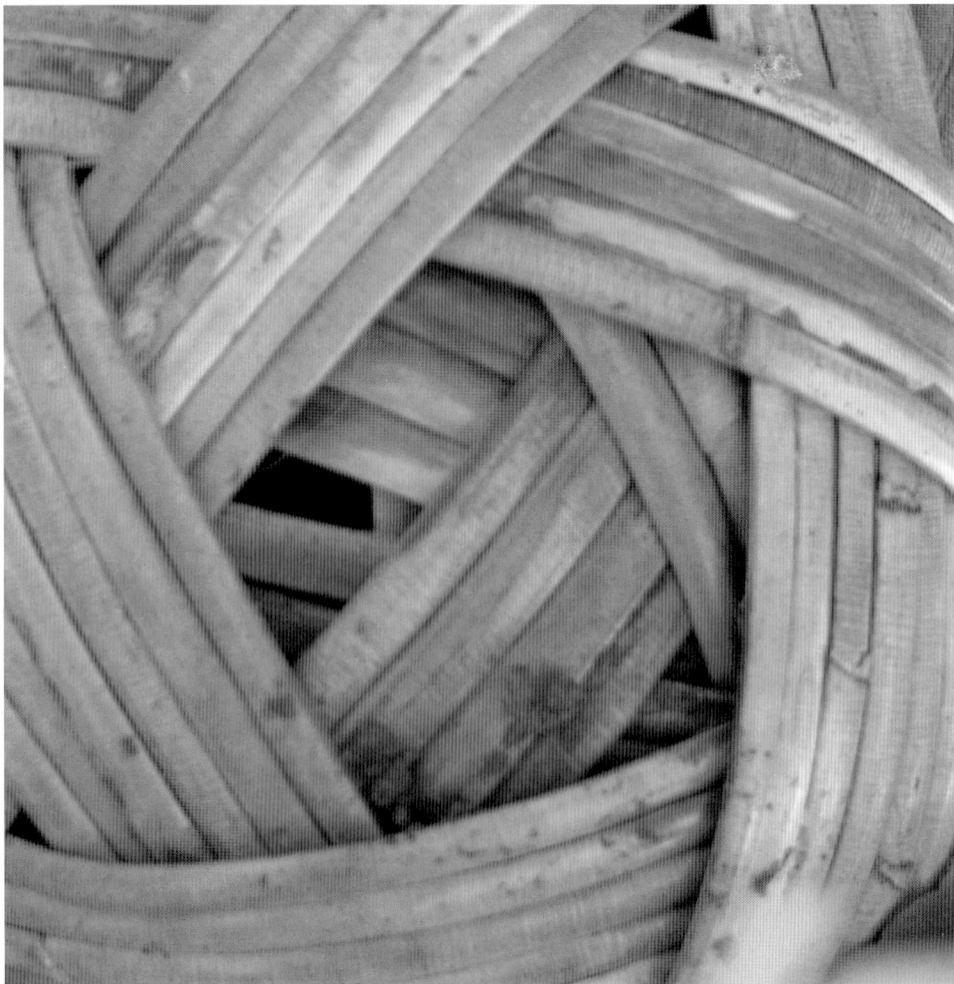

the sheer invisibility of an illness makes it more difficult to live with.

To avoid the pain that comes with all of this, and to find some explanation, I moved on. **Someone was to blame**.

Somehow, I don't know where and I don't know when, I must have been abused and this is how my psyche was responding. I had always been a sensitive little girl. Maybe that was it. Perhaps my mother and father had yelled too much at me. Maybe my brothers had bullied me too much.

My finger pointed everywhere. It didn't help. That is the funny thing about blame – it doesn't help you move, it just fuels the flames. I hadn't been abused, my parents did their best for me. And my brothers hadn't bullied me overly much. Eventually the finger pointed back to me. I was to blame. I knew that all along, of course. And this is where the story could end. Or start all over again. Chasing circles in my mind and getting nowhere.

Then there is the other offshoot of blame. Guilt. Whoever shoulders the blame has the added bonus of guilt. When you push blame onto somebody else you spread the feelings of shame. In the end, maybe that is what I wanted to do. If someone or something else was to blame it would have absolved me a little bit.

Something had to break the cycle. Something had to break the circle that revolved around me. I had to see beyond myself. I felt like a little girl whose protective balloon surrounding her had been pierced. I felt small, vulnerable and powerless. I had to do something.

And then the blessings began.

I began teaching students after their school day. I decided then and there that I would give them every bit of confidence I felt I lacked. I would support them, listen to them and work to have myself made redundant. I wanted their confidence to grow so that they would not need me. I saw their confidence grow and with theirs, mine grew. But something else was happening too.

One Saturday afternoon my rabbi spoke to us about *tikkun*. *Tikkun*, as I came to understand it, is a Hebrew word that embraces the concept of repair. I believe that my soul, or in Hebrew my *neshama*, has been in this world before. As my rabbi explained, my *neshama* was here to undergo *tikkun*.

Hey, hold on a moment. Let me get this straight. I have to go through the trials and tribulations of multiple sclerosis so that my neshama can repair itself? In other words, I am paying the price for somebody else's exciting life. What's the bet in a previous lifetime my *neshama* had been in the body of an Olympic gymnast and who knows what the gymnast got up to?

A bit simplistic perhaps but it had given me the jolt I needed. I started rethinking my reliance on blame.

'Okay, perhaps blame isn't the best explanation,' I thought. 'What about responsibility?'

And then came the big switch. What was my responsibility and how did multiple sclerosis tie in with this? Or put a bit differently, could multiple sclerosis be the key to my growing sense of responsibility?

My soul is the part of godliness within me. It is the most precious, the most rich and beautiful part. What a magnificent task it would be to beautify and enrich my *neshama*.

You see, I have this illness but it is only the beginning. How could I use the illness for my task? It didn't have to be ms. It could have been anything, another illness or whatever. When I was created, I was given a rare mixture of talents and gifts. How I use those talents and gifts is entirely up to me. Later on, I was given a little prod: multiple sclerosis.

Multiple sclerosis has been transformed. It has become no less frustrating, painful or hateful. But through it I have found my purpose, my direction. It is a purpose that elevates me beyond the illness and makes every day that I live with it, filled with the potential of meaning.

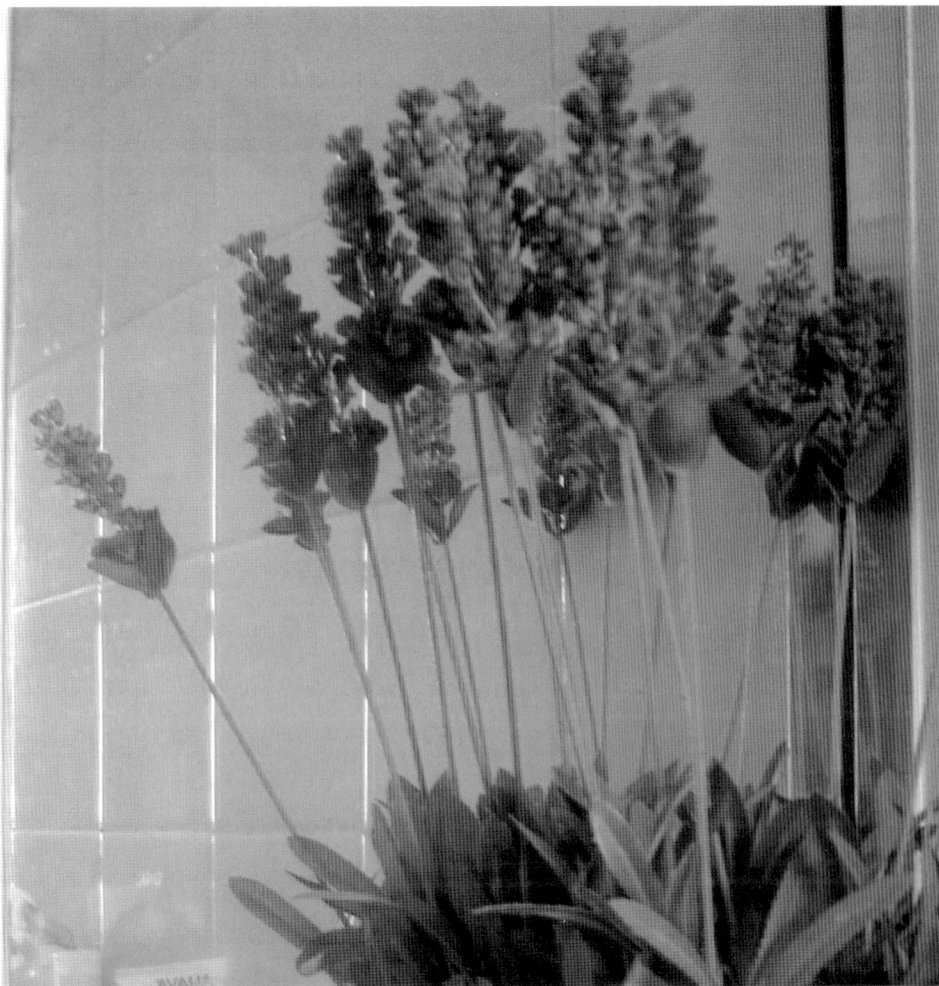

Victor Frankl wrote the most magnificent book, *Man's Search for Meaning*. Frankl survived the Holocaust and he writes of his experiences in Auschwitz. More than that, he writes of his survival and how he was able to find meaning even in that hell.

He wrote, '. . . and we had to learn ourselves and, furthermore, we had to teach the despairing men, that it did not really matter what we expected from life, but rather what life expected from us. We needed to stop asking about the meaning of life and instead to think of ourselves as those who were being questioned by life – daily and hourly . . . life ultimately means taking the responsibility to find the right answer to its problems and to all the tasks which it constantly sets for each individual.'

To take what J.F. Kennedy said, and jiggle it a bit: *Ask not what life has to offer you, but rather what you have to offer life.*

That puts me in the driver's seat. It is up to me to seek solutions for **my** life's problems. It changes everything. I am no longer a victim of my circumstances or my life. I do not suffer from the illness. I am not a victim. I live with it. And it is up to me to seek ways to fulfill what I believe is my purpose in life.

Once I found what my direction was, I was open to opportunities to fulfill my purpose. The people and opportunities presented themselves, and my eyes were opened to recognise them. But even more than that, I had the impetus and conviction to act on those opportunities. And that has made all the difference.

Oh, by the way, sadly, no one ever wins the blame game. Sorry!

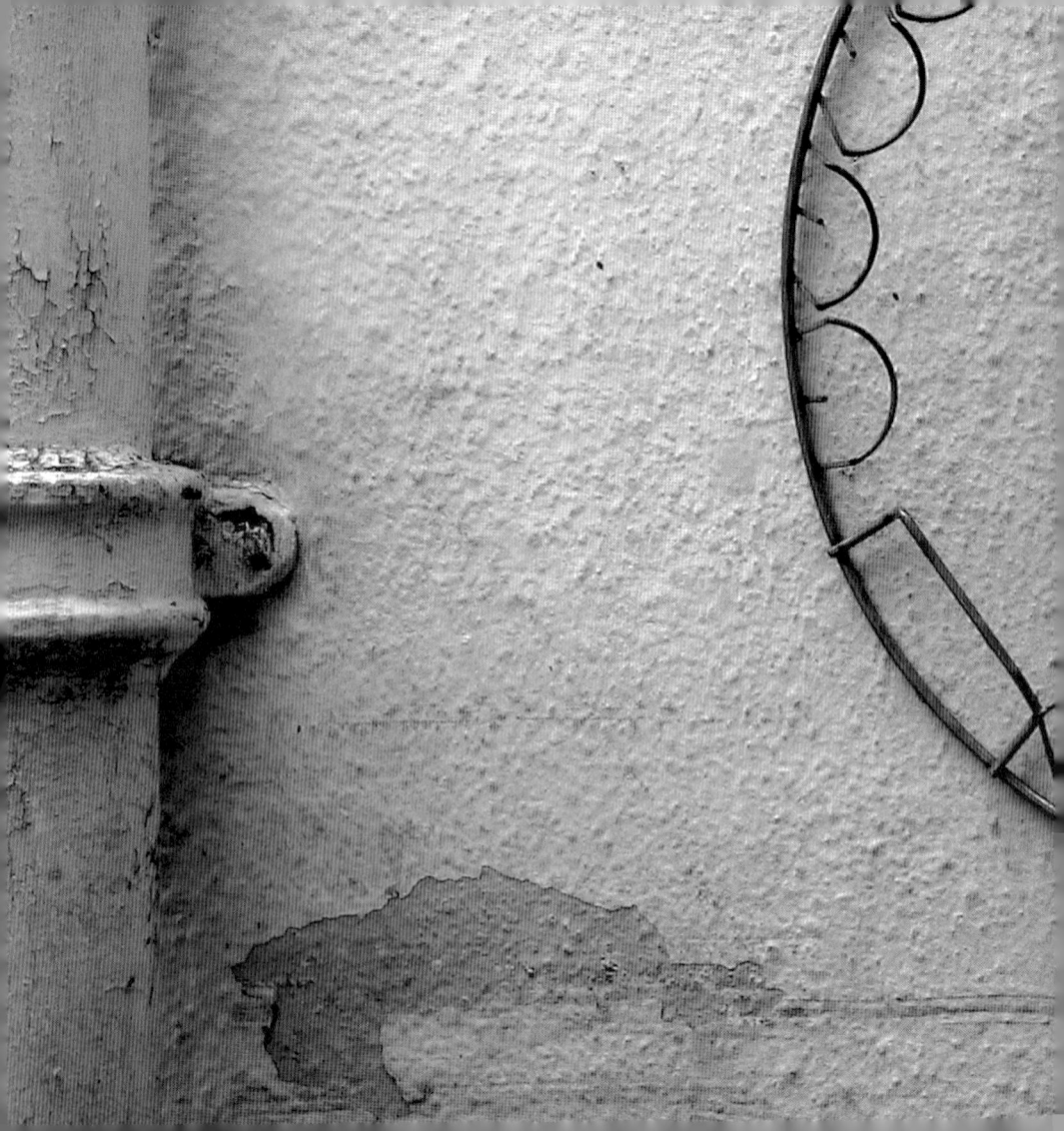

5. Seeking a Cure but Finding Healing

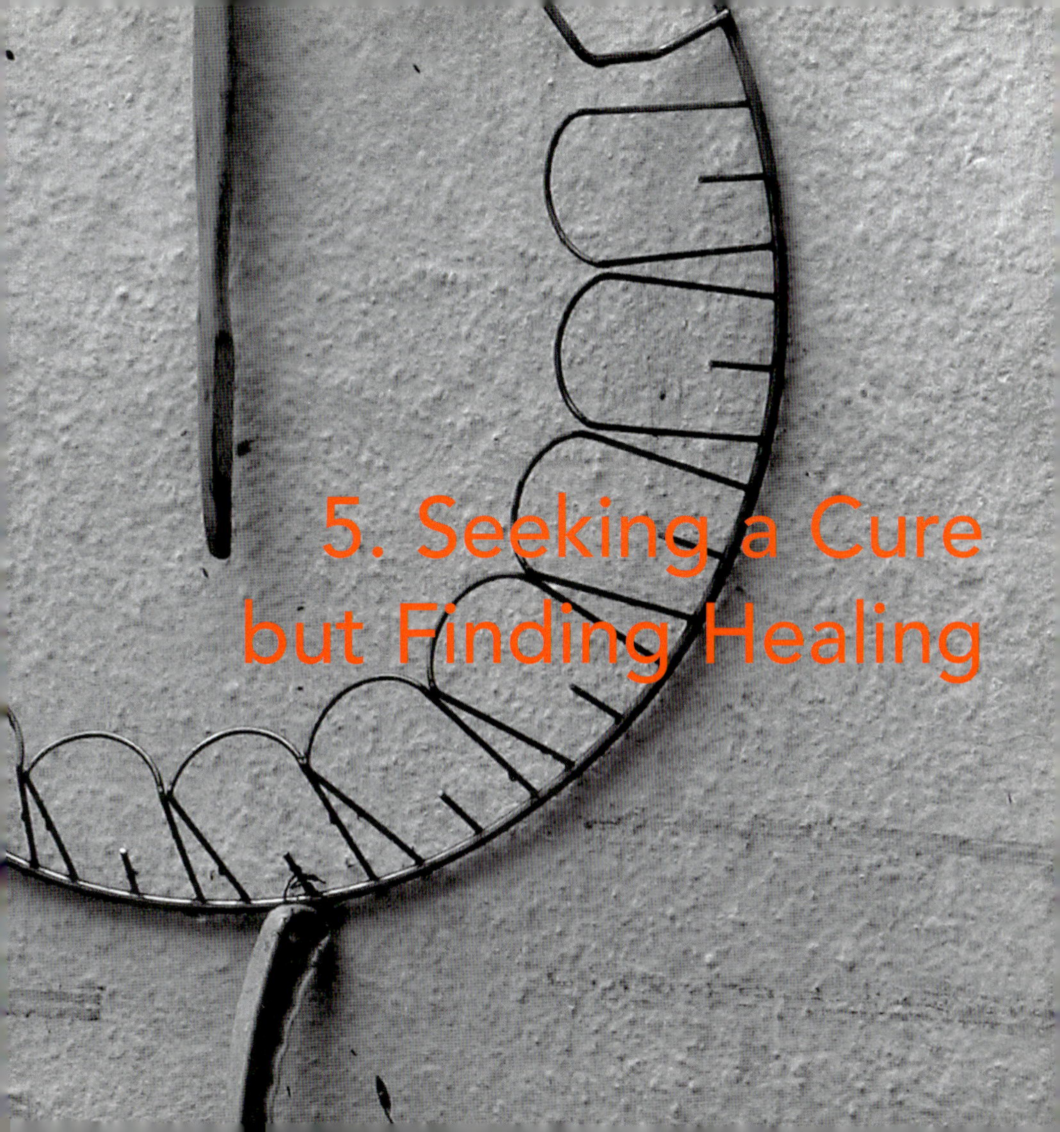

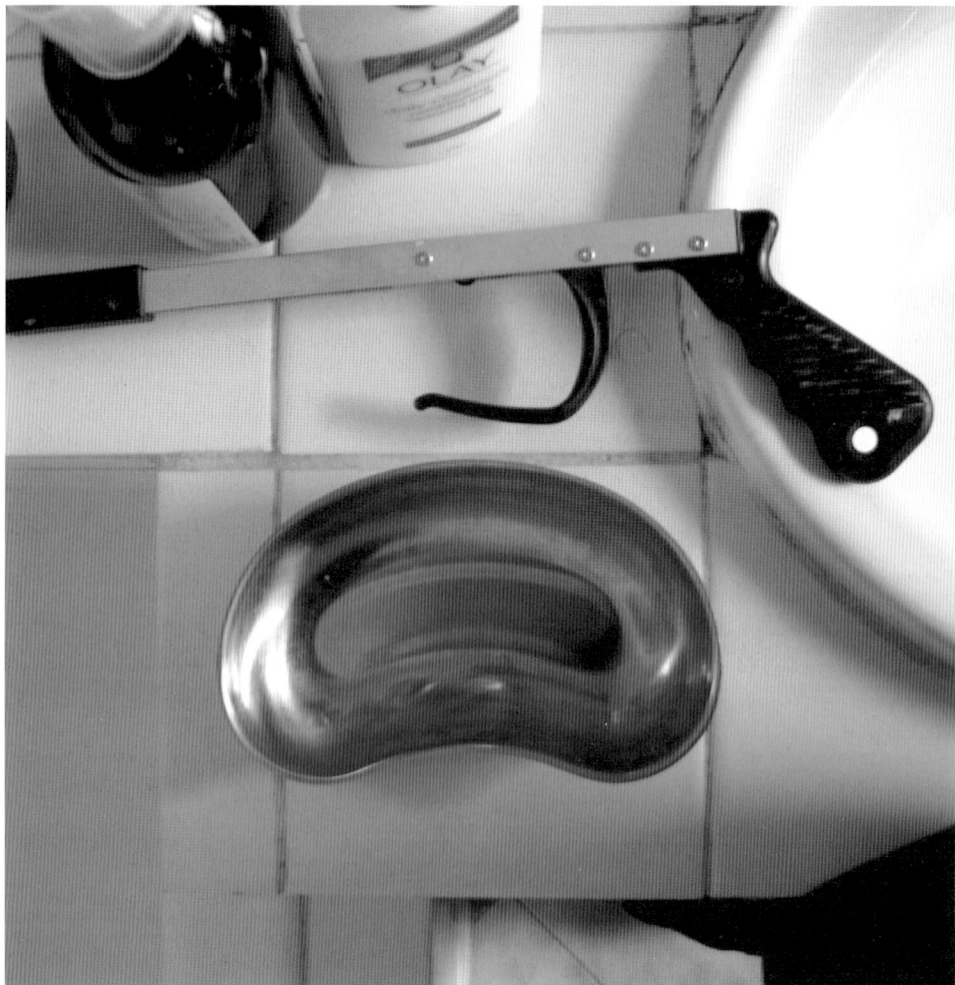

Living with a chronic illness that has no known cure, is frustrating and can sap you of your energy, both physical and mental.

Many people have written about the link between the way that you think and the way that your body responds. I have read books encouraging me to delve within myself to find the origins of my illness. You can become prey to purveyors of hope who have little idea of your own personal hell. Somewhere, deep within my psyche, nestled beneath years of living, lies The Answer. If I don't find It, either I have not looked hard enough or else I am lacking some exceptional quality. To the burden of living with the illness, add the burden of not being able to cure yourself. Pretty heavy.

I do not doubt that there are many people whose cancers mysteriously shrink. I do not doubt that thousands of people have been encouraged and given strength by their stories. But nobody has a magical formula that rids you of all illnesses. Even prayer seems to work for some people but not for others. The link between the mind and the body remains elusive to me.

I have heard the story told of children at boarding school who suffered terribly from homesickness. Perceptive caregivers listened to them and gave them 'homesick tablets'. Miraculously their homesickness was cured but what were they given? Sugar pills. And therein lies the fascinating conundrum of the placebo. Perhaps in the placebo lies the magical formula that can rid us of all illnesses. In any clinical trial, some people are given the drug being tested and others the placebo. That some people are helped by the drug is to be expected. But what fascinates me are those people that are helped by the placebo.

Norman Cousins writes of the placebo in his book *Anatomy of An Illness*: 'It is doubtful whether the placebo . . . would get very far without a patient's robust will to live. *For the will to live enables the human body to make the most of itself* [my italics] . . . the placebo, then, is an emissary between the will to live and the body. But the emissary is expendable. If we can liberate ourselves from tangibles, we can connect hope and the will to live directly to the ability of the body to meet greater threats and challenges.'

Theories are wonderful, but frustrating. Practically, what does this all mean? What do I have to believe in to rid me of my illness? All I want to do is to shout, 'I am sick of you, multiple sclerosis. I am tired of your tricks. Just go away!' Surely that should be enough?

I can either live with that frustration, that anger, or else I can try to change it. It is my choice. So the many books that have been written, somehow do not work for me. I can get angry with them for not understanding the complexity of what I have to live with, or else I can take what I can from them, and then close the books and look elsewhere for my answers. I can get angry with G-d for not curing me, or else I can acknowledge that I am not able to dictate to Him. G-d does answer prayers, but the answers are seldom simple. I have to look more deeply, forgive myself my lack of control and seek something far beyond a cure.

Bernie S. Siegel wrote the book, *Peace, Love, and Healing: The Path to Self-healing*, and it was this book that altered the way that I viewed myself and my life's journey. Siegel recognises the inherent problem of what happens if a person is unable to cure themselves of whatever illnesses may be ailing them. He writes 'Exceptional patients don't try not to die. They try to *live* until they die. Then they are successes, no matter what the outcome of their disease because they have healed their lives, even if they have not cured their diseases.'

As a surgeon, Siegel had the humility to write, 'If we doctors would admit our mortality, then we would find a way to succeed with even the sickest of our patients, sometimes simply holding their hands when they are frightened and in pain, other times helping them understand the meaning of their illness and how they can use it to experience life and love.'

This then became my quest: to find healing and in that healing, to experience life and love as never before.

I have had try to find a meaning beyond my illness. And in seeking meaning, I have been able to experience life and love in ways I might have overlooked. The first and most obvious love perhaps, is the love and respect I have found for myself. If I don't love my-self, respect myself, it is an uphill battle to retain the self-esteem that is vital for successful living. When your body reneges on you, it is like being a teenager all over again. With adult sensibilities, I have to get used to a new body image. I have to re-acquaint myself with a body that does not always do my bidding. I would like to ignore the parts of me that do not work. But how about taking a different route? What if I loved my body despite all its failings? Is it possible to look at my inabilities without frustration and anger?

A mother can look at her child with unconditional love. If her child has problems, she can feel indescribable sorrow and inde-scribable love all at the same time. And that is the type of love I need to have for myself. I have to cultivate that love, that unconditional love which is not dependent on a physical rating. Sometimes when I become too critical of myself, I stop myself. I have to tell myself to give myself a break. Be kind to myself. Think kindly. Speak kindly.

As my illness has progressed, I have become more dependent

on other people to enable me to do the simplest things in life. I now need help to get in and out of my bed. I need a nurse to help me get into and out of the shower. Without the solid bedrock of real care for myself, I would not be able to accept the love and care of others with grace. I cannot deny the frustration that comes from dependency. I cannot deny the fear that comes from my inability to take care of myself fully. There is no easy answer.

I have to look beyond myself. I have had to find a purpose in my life, a way in which I would still be able to contribute to society. I do not have children; I do not have a husband. In them I might have found a built-in purpose. Even that might not have been enough. Existential meaning I feel I have found in the concept of *tikkun* (repair – see chapter 3). I feel connected to the greater turnings of my soul and the souls of all those around me. But that is not bread-and-butter meaning. That comes with purpose. I write and I teach and I speak to groups. And I pray, 'Create a pure heart for me, O G-d, and a steadfast spirit renew within me.' (Psalms 51:12)

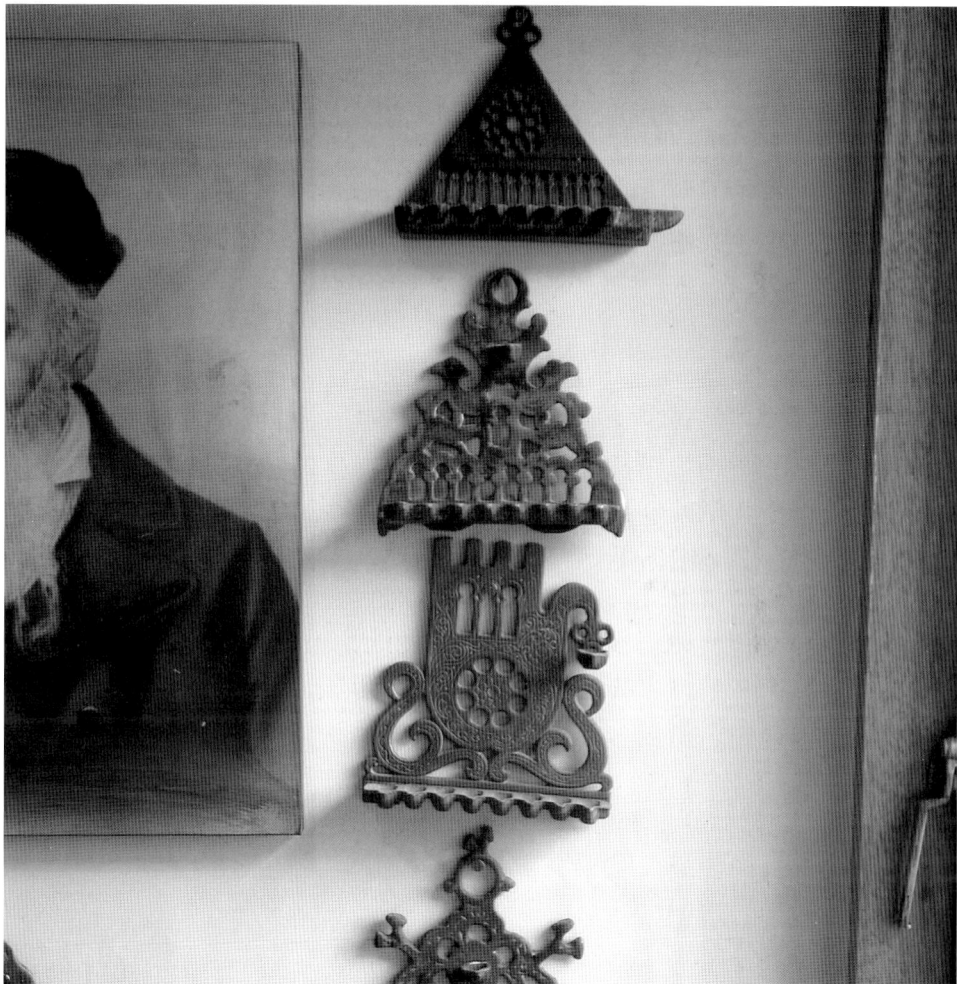

So it is with healing: The illness remains, with all its frustrations and pain, but it becomes a means to growth and spiritual calm. How does that happen? In as many ways as there are people in this world. I could no more tell you the exact moment or time that my illness, in itself, became inconsequential. Of course it predicates what I feel and is a part of me. I can't leave it behind and go on holiday, just for a break. But I believe that if it hadn't been multiple sclerosis it would have been something else.

A friend of mine, a recovering alcoholic, believes that he was chosen to be an alcoholic. But then all the means were put his way to recover. He had to take action to deal with his life. But once he had taken action, his life began all over again. All that his years of sobriety have taught him is the spirituality by which he must – has to – live. That spirituality has brought him humility, compassion, understanding and acceptance of all things, because all things have a purpose in life.

And so I believe it must be for me. The person I have become is greater than I was before I knew I had ms. It is useless to imagine what I could have been or done if I were not ill. Tempting perhaps, but ultimately painful and purposeless.

If I were told that a cure had been discovered for multiple sclerosis, I would be overjoyed. But in the meantime, what is stopping me from being overjoyed today? Nothing.

Absolutely nothing.

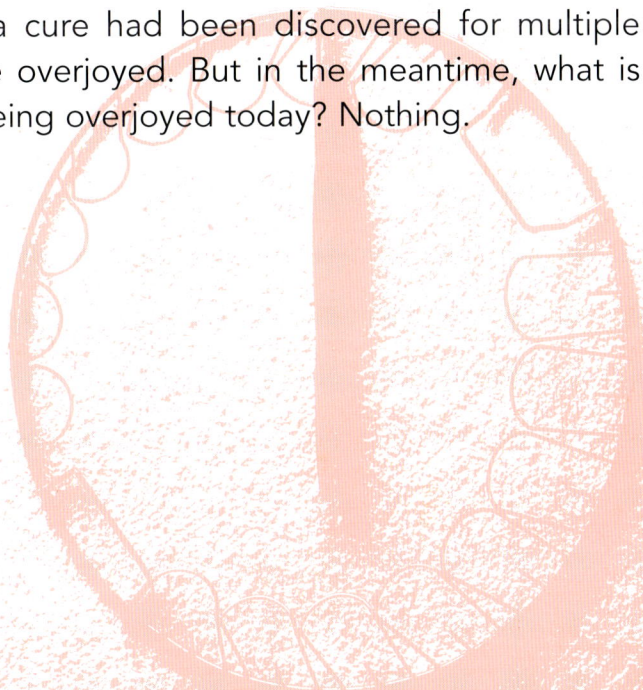

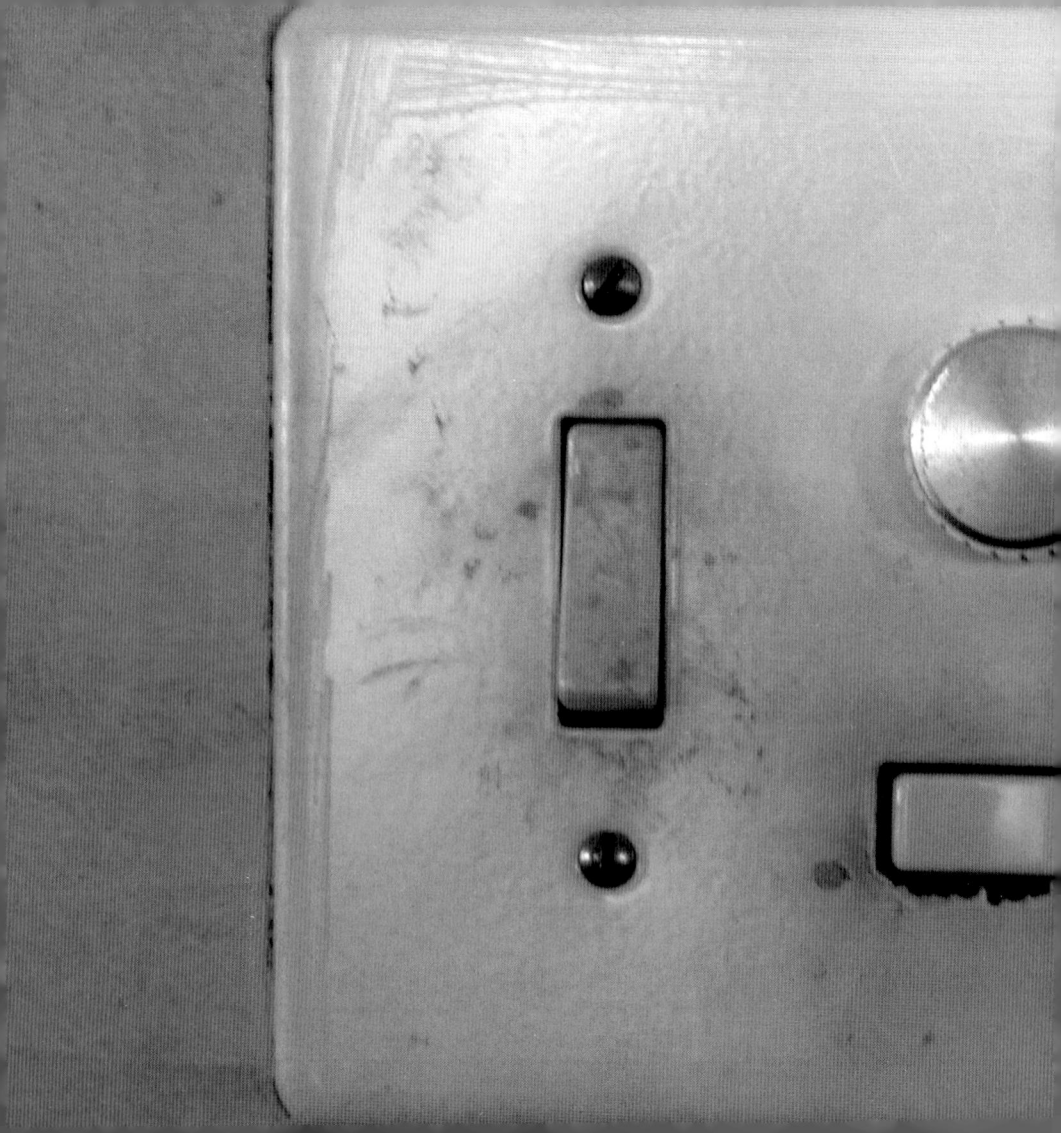

6. The Courage to Choose

One of the most exciting revelations that has come from living with my illness has been the realisation of my actual freedom to choose.

Spontaneity: the flexibility to change your mind, to do something just for the heck of it. To choose this or that direction, just because you can. The ultimate freedom of choice. But how many of us are able to use that freedom? Perhaps when we were younger, before job constraints or family concerns cramped that freedom.

Lord Peter Wimsey the hero of Dorothy Sayers' detective novels, has as his motto, 'As the Whimsy Takes Me'. I always wanted to adopt that motto. But I couldn't. I could never adopt the insouciant, carefree, devil-may-care approach to life. Just once I did go, 'as the whimsy took me'. I travelled Britain by train, stopping where I wanted, going where I chose. I trekked through Wordsworth's country in the mist and rain. I went to Stratford-upon-Avon, watched three plays and even got Jeremy Irons' autograph (three times!). I bought books on Sherlock Holmes

(I was a Sherlockian, member of the Sherlock Holmes Society of London). I walked the streets of London and sent postcards home to myself. 'Dear Me,' I wrote. My freedom to choose found its full expression in that holiday. Now my freedom is more circumscribed.

Viktor Frankl, in his book *Man's Search For Meaning*, writes, 'Everything can be taken from a man but one thing: the last of the human freedoms – to choose one's attitude in any given set of circumstances, to choose one's own way.'

That presents an exciting set of possibilities. Events, or sets of circumstance, have meaning because we give them meaning. So often we don't exploit our power to colour and shape our own world. It is how we choose to respond to events that makes the difference.

I am faced with a range of difficulties, living with multiple sclerosis. Pick any one of them – my difficulty in walking, my increased difficulty in writing (my signature keeps changing!),

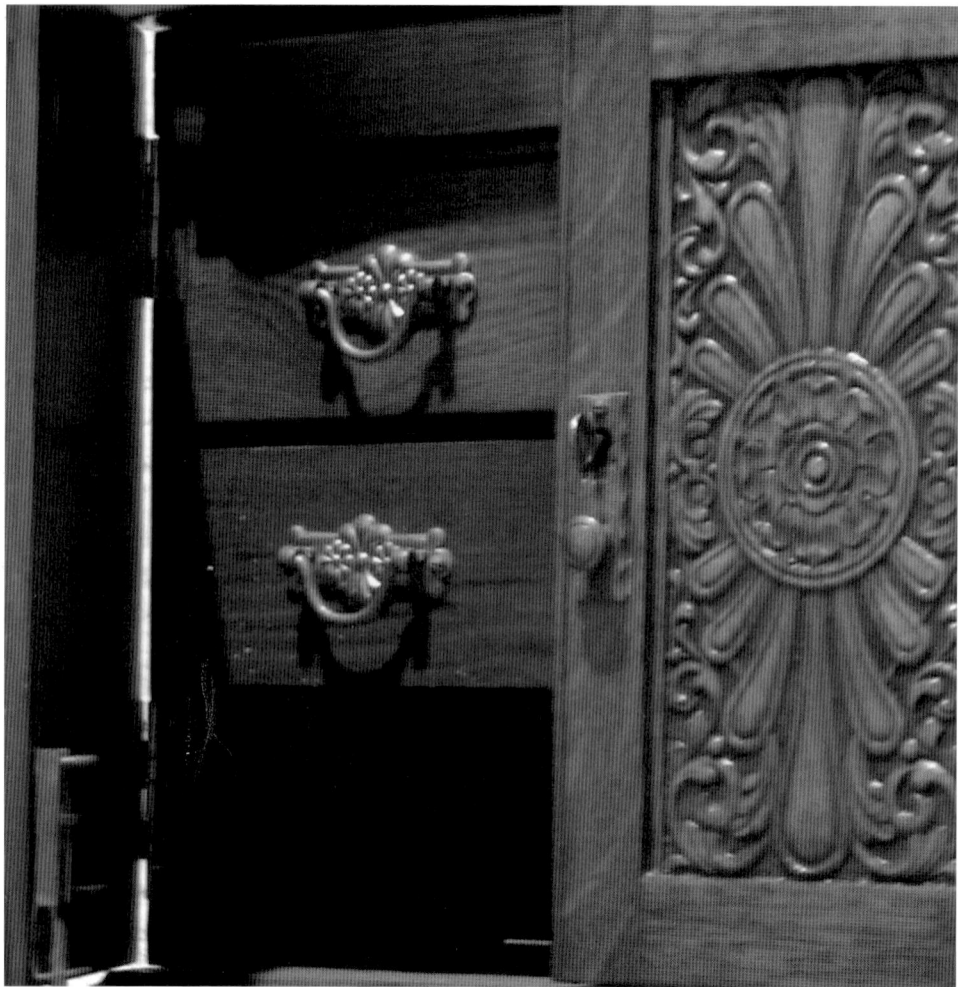

and problems with my bladder control. I need go into hospital for a cortisone treatment every few months. Those are the givens – no amount of positive thinking will change my reality. But how I shape my reality is up to me. I do not feel cheerful about my symptoms. I choose, however, to look at my own set of circumstances and at my life with a positive tinge.

My bladder has not been behaving itself of late. Incontinence is one of the more troubling symptoms of multiple sclerosis. It can be managed of course, as most of these symptoms can be. But just sometimes, my bladder does not behave. Or perhaps I don't react fast enough. When my bladder whispers, I have to respond quickly. I have to get up, get onto my scooter, go to the loo. Sometimes when I ignore the whisper, I find myself sitting on my chair and my bladder just lets go.
Not again.
Here I am sitting in a puddle of pee with nobody nearby to assist me. Then I give myself a choice: Either I sit and wait for somebody to come to help me or else I get onto my scooter and help myself. I make the choice and get onto my scooter.

Having made the decision to clean myself up, I encourage myself. There is nobody around to praise my decision. There is nobody about to cheer me on and to advise me. So I do it myself. Aloud.

'Right Lauren, go get a towel and mop up the mess. Great! Now, wipe the chair. Fine! Now I think that you should get changed into your pyjamas. It doesn't matter that it is so early but they are much easier to put on . . .' And so I manage, with self-esteem intact.

Irina Filatova, with whom I was privileged to work, quotes a Russian proverb. Very loosely translated it goes, 'When you have no choice, you become brave.' I smile at that proverb because it is only half true. Given the choice I would not have this illness, but once I have it, I do choose to become brave. I do choose to paint my world with yellows and blues and purples. There are many terrible situations in life – there is a time for mourning and a time for grieving. However, one can get bogged down in misery and self-pity. Of course it is difficult, but it is vital to find the strength to choose to seek a way out of the darkness to the light. It is not easy to choose your own perspective. It takes courage and perseverance.

One of the other symptoms I live with is what I call, 'ms rage'. One particular Saturday, my mind went spinning: My earning potential had been severely curtailed. And there were so many things I needed to take care of financially and there were so many things that are so tempting to buy. If only I had another couple of thousand rand', I reasoned, 'everything would be fine'.

And then there is that damned heat. I cannot bear it when it is hot. My muscles seem to melt. I can't think clearly. The anger inside me bubbles like molten lava.

And then it erupts.

I yell at anyone who is nearby. I dredge up memories and fling accusations. Irrational, certainly. But full of pain.

Feelings of helplessness, frustration and vulnerability are eclipsed by my eruption of anger. And afterwards my feelings of shame. I'm sorry, but I didn't mean to yell at you. I'm sorry.

So where is the choice? I am entitled to my feelings, surely? It is understandable that in my situation I should feel frustration and anger. I can't be blamed for that, can I? It's natural.

But of course I can choose. Not when I am in the midst of an outburst of rage, but just before.

I remember when I was in hospital for a cortisone treatment. Intravenous cortisone is used to dampen down the effects of a relapse in multiple sclerosis. In many ways it is a wonder drug but it plays havoc with one's emotions.

I was expecting a visit. And they were late. They knew how I depended on visits. Damn. I held the telephone next to me and picked up the hand set. I was ready to phone them, give them a piece of my mind. Then I stopped.

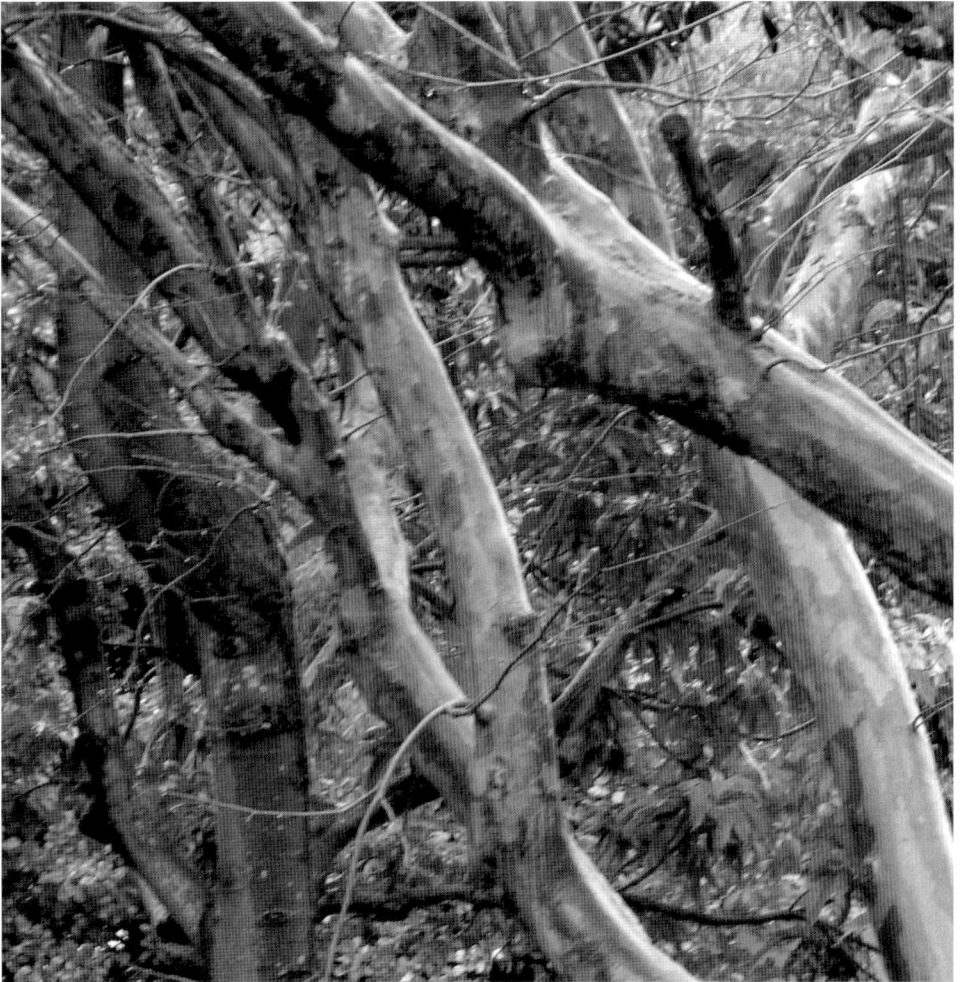

And gave myself a choice. I could phone, but I knew the conse-quences. I would phone in anger. I would justify myself, but then they would. I would yell and we would all end up feeling terrible.

And if I didn't phone? What could I do to calm myself down? Stop the train of thought that would inevitably end in a train smash. Have a cup of tea, which always worked to soothe me. Support myself, encourage myself. Read or listen to music or watch television. It worked. I didn't phone and felt magnificent.

Anger is something we all live with and it is not confined to any particular illness or circumstance. Anger drags us back in time, and past slights and annoyances come back to fuel the flames. Sometimes, it is an unconscious choice to get into a rage. And let it control us.

We feel justified in our anger. It is what we do with it that is para-mount. I have found that if I can acknowledge my anger before it erupts, I can re-establish my freedom of choice. Sometimes I cannot and I have to live with the consequences. Sometimes there are emotional triggers like vulnerability, frustration and helplessness that are difficult to recognise. Sometimes we feel we aren't being listened to and our opinions amount to nothing, anyway. Acknowledge those feelings and the anger dissipates. It is a matter of choice, but sometimes it takes courage to face our vulnerability. Then we can become our own loving 'parent' again. We can comfort ourselves, acknowledge our feelings and validate ourselves.

This is where the real control rests. With that control comes freedom. I may not be able to go 'as the whimsy takes me', but neither do I have to go 'as my rage takes me.'

And that is real freedom.

7. Surprised by Joy

Disclaimer: the following chapter might be disturbing to someone who has lost their sense of humour, or to someone who thinks they might have lost their sense of humour. If concerned, please consult a friend (preferably at 3 a.m.).

It seems so simple, but I know that laughter and a sense of humour have been my saving grace. Not that everyone appreciates my humour. I remember meeting a woman who had recently been diagnosed with multiple sclerosis. Along with the support I hoped I gave, her family and I had a good chuckle. She did not join in. Wrong time and wrong jokes. She was very astute – she saw that I used my humour as a coping mechanism.

And as a mask.

Timing is everything. I remember speaking to a fellow ms'er (someone living with multiple sclerosis) when I was first diagnosed and remarking that having ms wasn't so bad, anyway. 'Don't tell me you are a Pollyanna,' was her rejoinder. I did not find that funny. But then, I found little to laugh at.

Learning to live with a new, painful situation is like wearing-in a badly fitting pair of shoes. It's uncomfortable and often one feels self-conscious. And you cannot take the damned shoes off. The blisters are painful and you feel pinched. But as you wear them in and as you adjust to their shape, it's easier to look around you without a grimace. The shoes may never become fully comfortable, but you develop calluses where blisters once were. And you learn to laugh to smooth over the pain.

I enjoy my own quirky sense of humour. But there is something more to laughter. Laughter helps to restore a sense of balance. It is so easy to become self-absorbed, to lose your sense of perspective. It is like being afraid of the shadow monster under your bed at night. Switch on the light and the monster disappears. Laughter sheds light and spreads warmth throughout your being.

Much research is being done on the positive physiological effects of laughter. Laughter is said to boost your immune system, lower your blood pressure, chase away depression and relax you. Norman Cousins was being treated for ankylosing spondylitis, a painful arthritic disease, when he found that the treatment that he was being given was not helping him. So, he shut himself in a room and watched comedy after comedy. The Marx Brothers and many others cheered him. He laughed and laughed. Belly laughs. Was he happier? Clearly, but what was miraculous was that his illness went entirely into remission. His book, *Anatomy of an Illness,* was published in 1979 and he writes of the healing qualities of laughter.

I used to watch illicit copies of a British comedy television show in my student days in the 1980s. *Not the Nine o'clock News* was banned by the SABC. Its anarchic political humour did not tickle their funny bone. It did tickle mine. I remember going through a particularly bleak time soon after my diagnosis. I listened to a scratchy audio tape of the programme which I begged a friend to send me. I just needed to laugh. I now have a DVD of selections of *Not the Nine O'Clock News.* When I'm feeling blue, I put on the DVD and I am transported back in time and I laugh and giggle. I can repeat most of the skits verbatim.

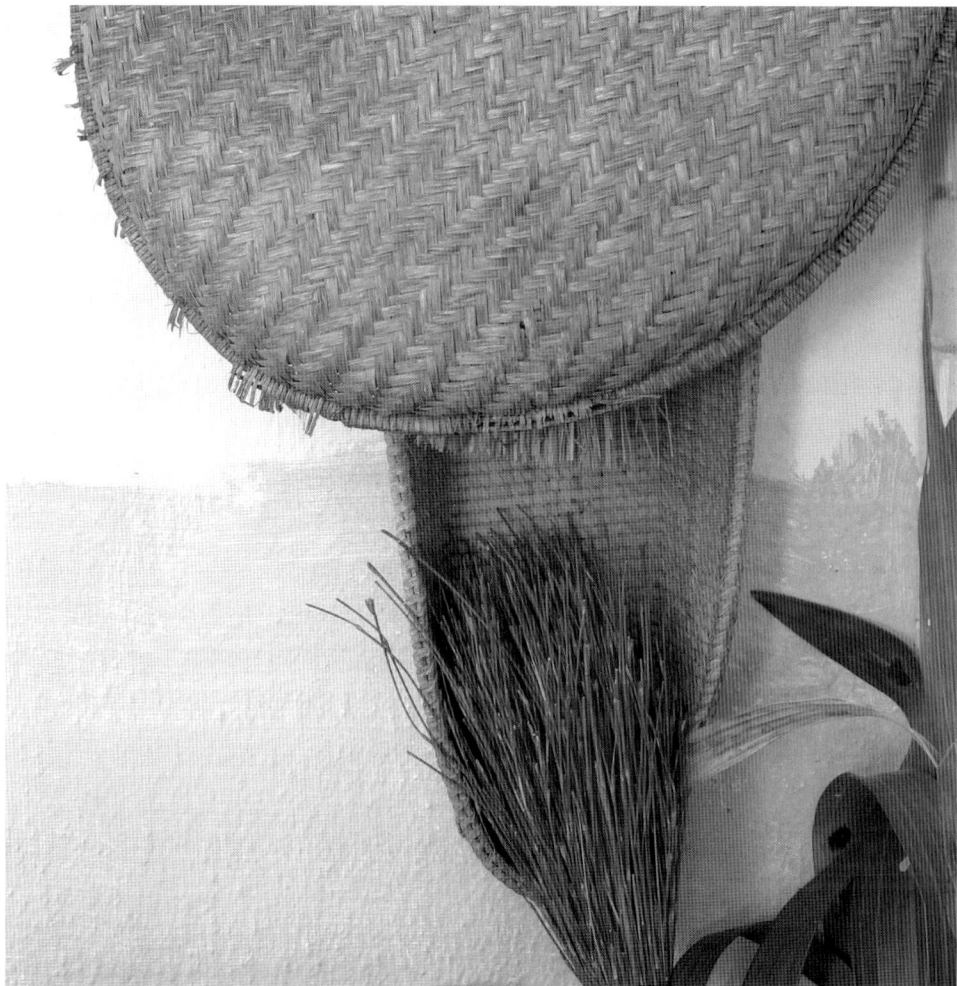

I feel great. Again I am faced with the question, 'So, am I going to be cured as Norman Cousins was?' I believe that Norman Cousins was healed and curing came as a byproduct of the healing.

There is something rich and spiritual about laughter. Laughter can be destructive, can be used to diminish and hurt someone. But when used wisely, laughter can be powerful. I have books of cartoons drawn during the Second World War. Cartoonists are astute observers of society and can encapsulate the mood and emotions of people living through difficult times. I compare the British cartoons of Pont and Fougasse with those of Russian cartoonists and I can see the differences in each society's experience and understanding of war. The one is phlegmatic and the other bloody and brutal. But there is a common thread that passes through all of the cartoons. Laughter. They are drawn to elicit a smile or a chuckle. When I get the morning paper, I quickly turn to the editorial page. 'Wonderful', I think if there is a Grogan cartoon on the page. Tony Grogan has the uncanny ability to tease out the laughable from a sometimes pitiful situation.

And that is the essence of the healing power of laughter.

When G-d told Abraham and Sarah that they were going to have a son, they laughed. Sarah laughed out of disbelief. She was too old, surely it could not be. Abraham laughed out of pure joy. What a surprise, even though he was so old, he was going to have a son. So important was their laughter that their son, Isaac, was named for it. Isaac comes from the Hebrew word meaning 'to laugh'. It is the laughter of Abraham that heals.

We can take a painful situation and find laughter in it. It does not change the situation, but we can look at it from a new perspective. Sometimes we are so immersed in pain, that the thought of finding joy seems remote. But even in our deepest despair a shaft of light may shatter the darkness when, 'surprised by joy'[1] we may find some consolation and healing in laughter.

[1] William Wordsworth wrote the sonnet entitled *Surprised by Joy* some time after the death of his daughter, Catherine, who had died at the age of 4. It is a beautiful evocation of grief and healing.

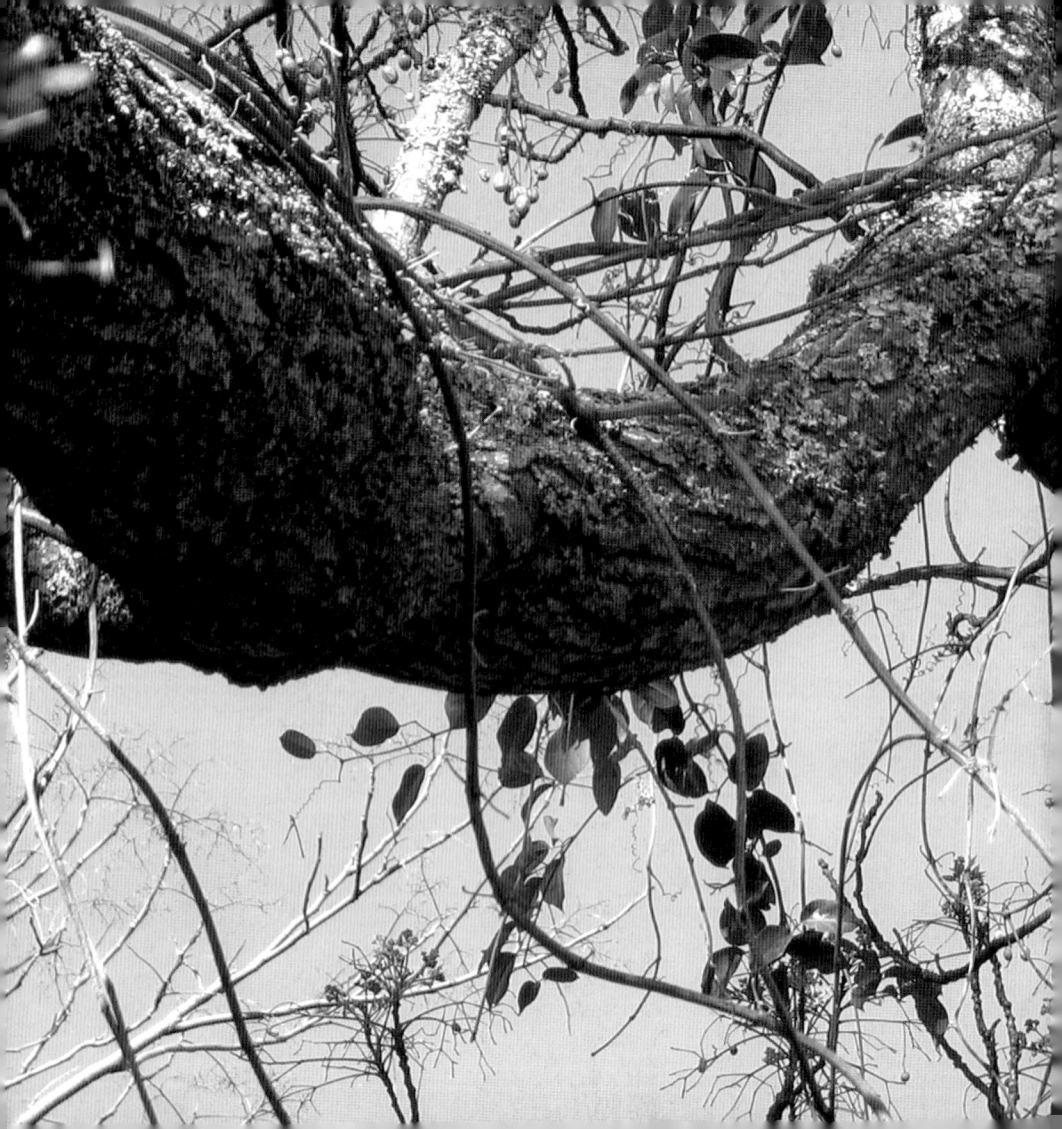

8. A Touch of Eternity

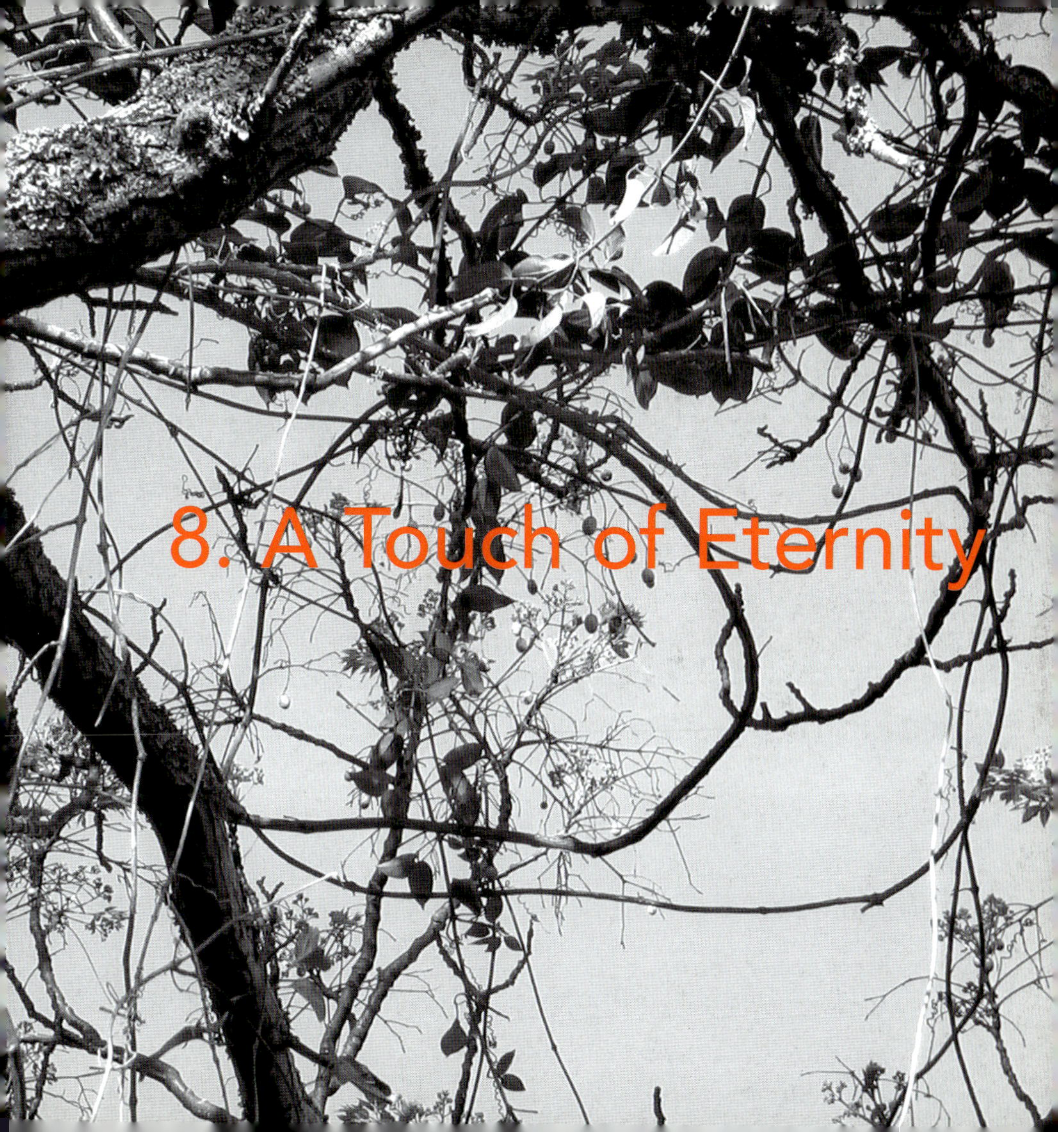

Sometimes people tell me how fortunate I am to be able to put my feelings into words. I am fortunate; I am blessed. But I cannot take full credit. When someone comments on how lovely my hands are, I tell them that my Granny gave them to me. Indeed, her gloves fit my hands perfectly. So when people say I have a way with words, I can only shrug and say, 'My *Bobba* (grandmother) was a poet, you know.'

'What is her name?' my Zeida (grandfather) asked my delighted parents when I was born.
'Lauren? Beautiful name, but what is her real name?'
He left, thought a bit and came up with the answer.
'Laya. We will name her for my late grandmother. A strong woman, the matriarch who kept our family alive in times of bitter cold and hunger in Latvia.'

So I am named Laya in Hebrew, named with pride after my ancestor who was strong and courageous. The abilities of my life have been passed on through generations. What I do with them, how I take the mixture and add a dash of personality, is my job.

And therein lies the excitement and the mystery of living!

Part of the mystery is the people we meet. I have met people who, for their own reasons, have tried to push me down. All of us have met people, and been friendly with people, who see the world differently from the way we do. I have felt betrayed and have cried and questioned myself. But I have tried not to keep those people with me. I have carried the hurt, but in the end I have tried to put it down. I have too much to carry without that pain. But sometimes the pain and the hurt lingers like a low drone in my ears. It is then that I am grateful for the symphony of my life that drowns out the drone.

I will never forget the chance encounters with two women on two different trains. The first woman held my hand as I wept and cried. She never knew me and never knew why I was so upset. I had just heard that my dearest childhood friend, Naomi, had been killed in a car accident. I said nothing and neither did she, but she comforted me. I met the second woman on my grand tour of England by train. I was alone, as was she, and both of us had just seen a play in Stratford-upon-Avon. Full of excitement, we shared our love of the theatre. We discussed the play, and the brilliance of the actors. And the common thread? I was alone on both occasions, made a brief contact which somehow made an impact, but did not change the course of my life. When I felt alone, two strangers reached out and touched me. They gave me a part of themselves which enriched me, and I wonder whether the part of myself I entrusted with them was, in turn, enriching. I believe so.

Bernie Siegel writes about the healing quality of love. All the people that have ever meant anything to me have given me love in varying shades and tones. More than that, they have enabled me to give them love. I believe that healing comes in the giving of love and care, and, importantly, in its acceptance. My professor, Apollon, once said to me, 'I love you and I like you.' He was the man who set me on my path of healing. The work I did at the Centre for Russian Studies was wondrous – and not just because it was intellectually stimulating. I worked in an atmosphere of love. I worked harder and I learnt more because

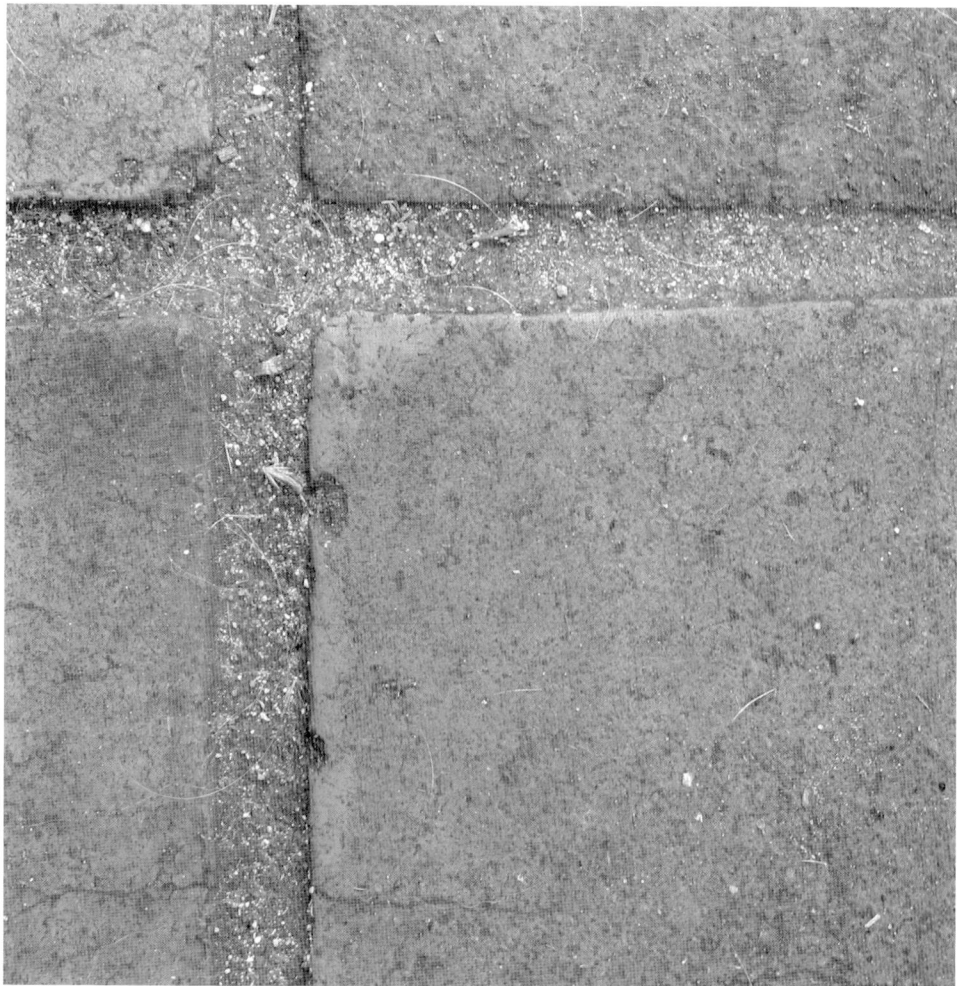

of that love. The time spent there plays in the leitmotif of my sustaining life-symphony. Even when I was advised to leave the university, a crushing blow, I was sustained by that love and care and respect.

At a time when the stuffing seems to be knocked out of you, it is vital to gather around you people who affirm who you are. Give you stability. My parents have always stood by me and given me the strong base from which I can grow.

But in addition I was lucky, at that time, to have my friend Owen to remind me of my own self-worth. He was the best of friends, a mentor. I believe that we meet the people we are meant to meet, at a time we are meant to meet them. We cannot fulfill our purpose in life without them and they cannot fulfill their purpose without us. The day after I met Owen he sent me an e-mail: 'Somewhere in time and space we have come together again.' Ours was a friendship of the soul. I knew him in the final five years of his life and I believe that he needed me to help complete his life's journey. And I needed him to help me progress in mine.

We have so many facets of ourselves to explore, and different friends help us to explore different facets. Sean is a great friend of mine. We seldom see each other, but we speak to each other every day. Both of us live with different chronic illnesses. A connection, a bond has been forged over the years. We do not share the same illness, but we strive to make sense of it all. Through our friendship I have known the frustration of not being able physically to help a friend. I can do nothing to make his illness better, but I can listen and empathise. Living with a chronic illness can be intensely lonely. I need to feel part of the world's movement. Although I feel isolated at times, I need to know that I have a role to play in life's turning. Apollon once said to me that it is good to feel needed. We all need to feel important, to feel that we matter. I matter in Sean's life, and he matters in mine.

It is the realisation of your role and place in the intricate dance of life that gives meaning to relationships, no matter how lasting or fleeting. And an appreciation of that intrinsic quality of love, brings healing.

I have yet another love that is as uncomplicated as it is pure and real. I do not doubt it and I do not doubt that it is given with a fulsome desire to please. He loves many and greets them all with abandon. He runs to give them gifts, shouting his joy to see them. If he hasn't seen one of his loves, he does not forget him, or her. Even after years of separation he greets him with as much joy as if he had seen him just the day before. Strange, because if he had been separated from one he loves for even a few hours, his joy is just the same.

Robert Browning wrote a magnificent poem, *His Last Duchess*. I read that poem and shiver. Jealousy and anger are wrapped up together when he sees the smiles his duchess lavishly bestows on others. But if I were to write a poem about my dearest friend, there would be no jealousy. Only gratitude because I have learnt so much about love, and the giving of love from my friend, Fred – Professor Fred Huggins DHH, my beautiful golden retriever.

Fred is the greatest healer without knowing it. Touch is extremely important, and Fred thrives on hugs. So do I. He and I share a sense of humour, which is fortunate. When I feel glum, he knows how to cheer me up. I know that I can tell him anything, and he will never repeat it. The ultimate in confidentiality. He accepts me without question, doesn't try to change me. He shows concern with a look and stays close to me for mutual re-assurance. I cannot quantify his healing ability. I cannot walk better because of him. But I know he dislikes ms as much as I do. He said in his own book, *Fred at Your Service, Ma'am*, that if he ever met ms he would pee on his foot. Good boy, I know you would.

My mother has always said that life is a confidence trick. When you feel confident, you learn. You live better when you have confidence in yourself. You make better decisions when you have confidence in yourself. You attract the people that will help you grow. And you attract love when you feel yourself able to give love. When you love and are loved, you come closer to the Source of all healing. There is something spiritual in the healing quality of love.

For love is a powerful energy that never dissipates – moreover, it tantalises you with a touch of eternity.

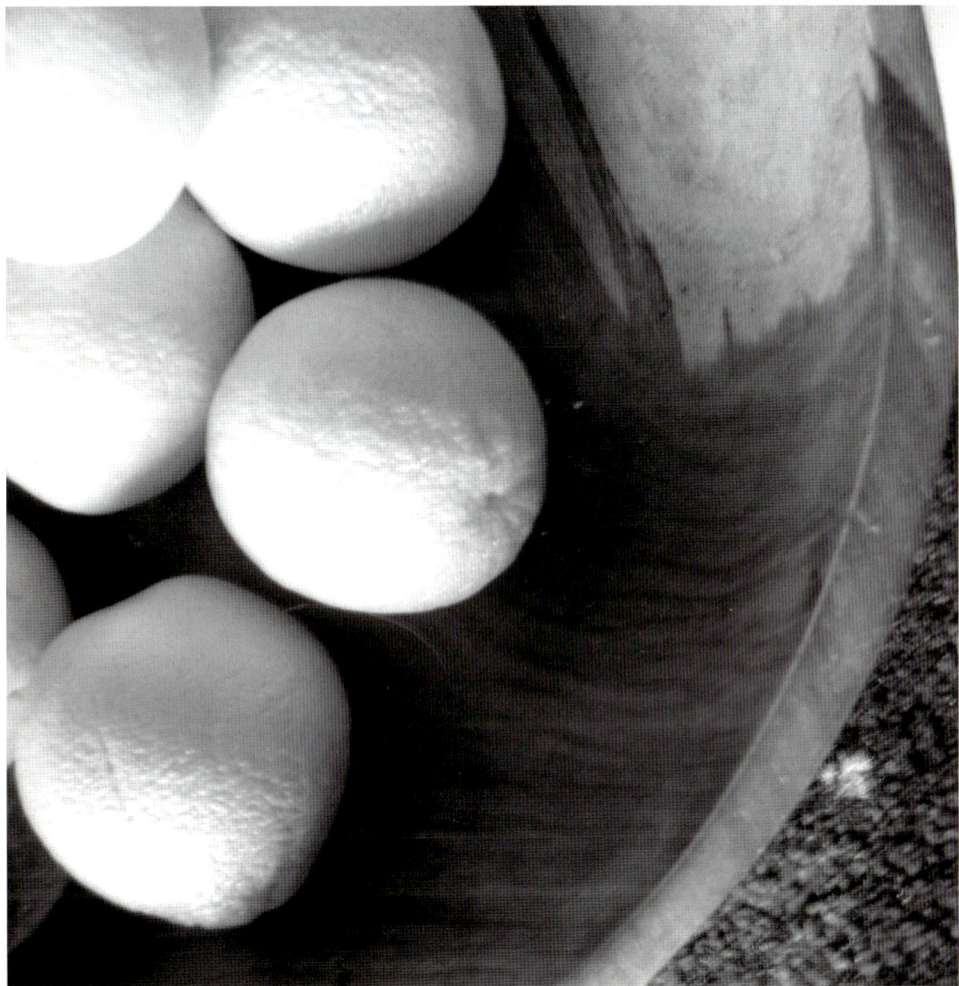

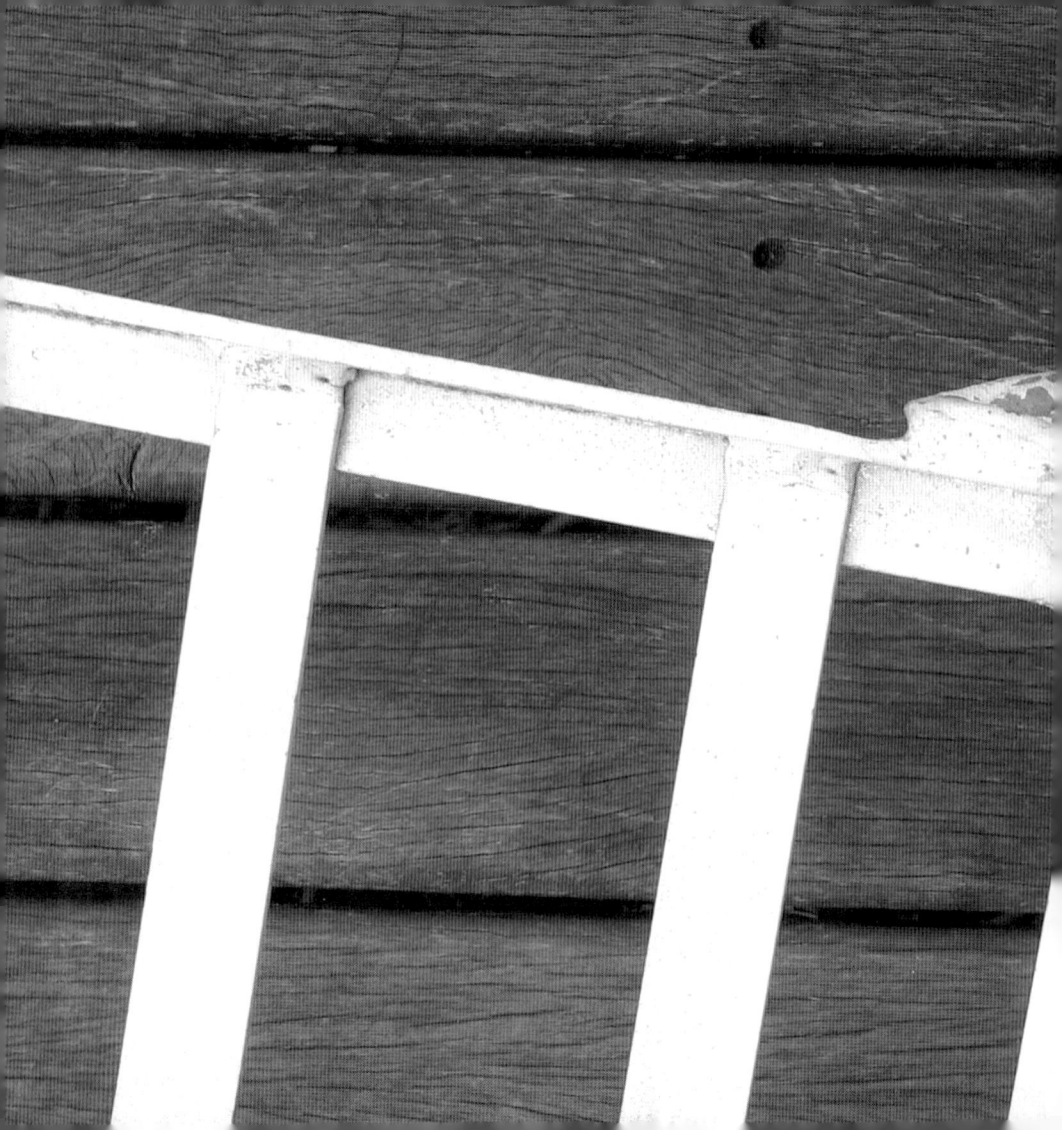

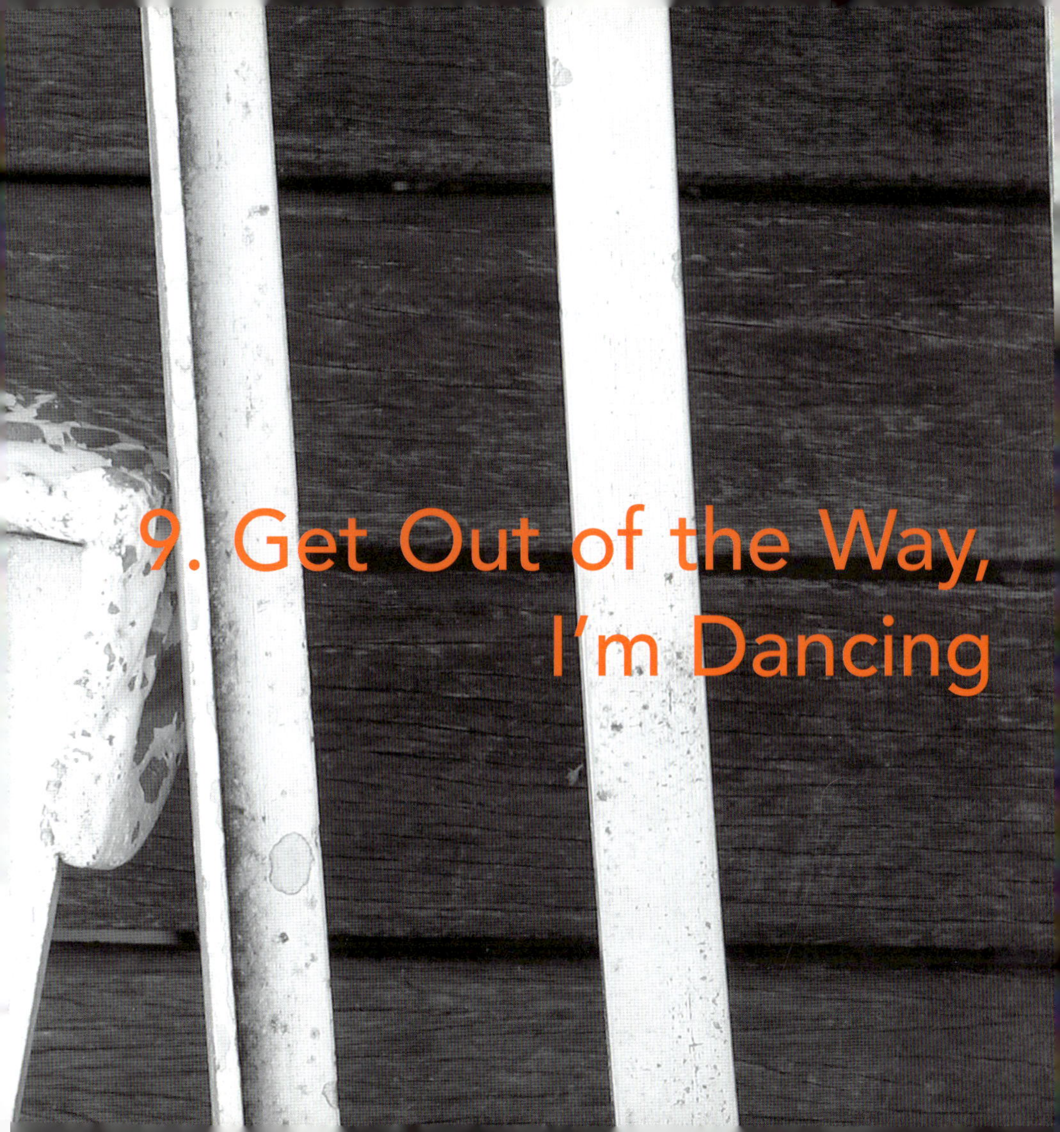

9. Get Out of the Way, I'm Dancing

The research laboratory in which I worked when I lived in Israel, was on the same floor as the psychiatric wards. Every now and then a patient would wander into our offices. One young man in particular would stroll through for a regular chat. He had an open, sweetly smiling face that held a certain innocence. I never knew why he was in hospital. He did not tell me. One day he came in holding a guitar. He sat on the floor and began to play.

The music was sweet, uncomplicated. To the musically trained ear, which I do not possess, it might have been discordant. You see, he played a guitar which had one string missing. He clearly enjoyed playing and strummed with a confident air. And I looked on and listened with amazement. His playing has remained, for me, a metaphor for life.

Psychologically, the young man did not possess a full complement of strings. But he made do with what he had, and made music. Perhaps it was discordant, but not to me and clearly not to him. To my reckoning, people around me appear to have everything. They can walk, perhaps run. They may be married, perhaps they have children. Maybe they have a job, and they can buy the things they need. They can buy luxuries and can go away on holiday. Maybe they have a partner they can talk and chat to and laugh with. When Valentine's Day comes, there is somebody to give chocolates to. And somebody who sends them roses. But seldom do we see the complete picture.

Practically, who of us live with a full complement of strings, lacking nothing? I remember once being asked, what did I see in the future for myself? That was a difficult question. I felt at the time that my life was falling apart. I had just finished my Honour's degree and was under therapy, trying to figure out what my newly diagnosed illness meant to my life. It does not matter how and it does not matter why, but there are few of us that have not felt ourselves sinking lower into the depths. Future? I felt I had no future. But I asked questions, I pushed my beliefs and made demands on myself that made me face my fears. Fears of intimacy and failure. Fears of dependency. And as time has passed, and my physical abilities have diminished, I remember with gratitude the young man who played his guitar

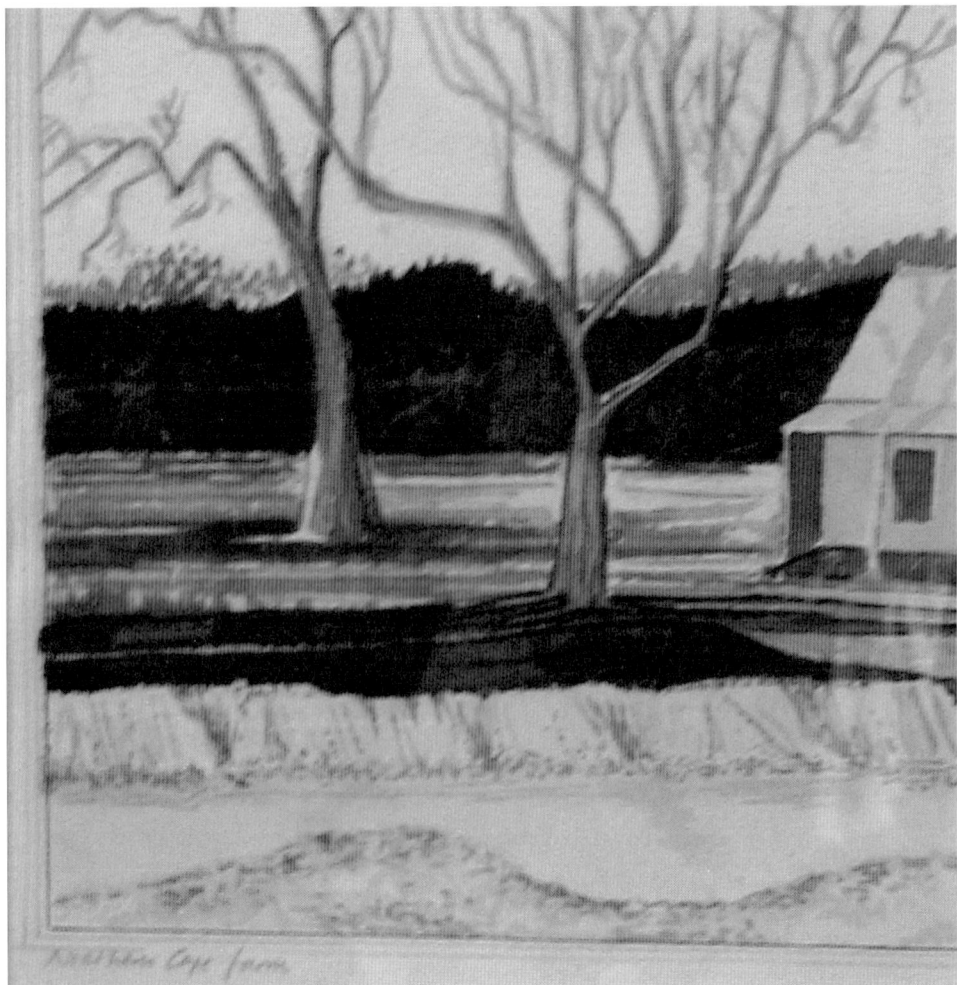

North Pelham Cape Farm

with one string missing. He taught me a valuable lesson: The trick, you see, is to learn to make music with what I do have.

Recently, I was invited to a wedding – it was meaningful and joyful. After the ceremony, we moved to the reception room and waited to greet the bride and groom. As they walked in, the music started playing. The women danced in a circle around the bride, and the men around the groom. We sang and clapped and danced – the atmosphere throbbed with excitement. I sat on the periphery, bouncing up and down on my scooter in time with the music. Then I was beckoned into the centre of the circle of women and sat, on my scooter, next to the bride. The women danced around us and I was included in the heady joy. The bride held my hand and looking into her face I saw her amazement. Her face glowed with awe and I basked in the reflection of her glory.

I remember how I used to join in the dancing. I was never light on my feet, but dancing in a circle of women, who ever noticed? An enthusiastic dancer, I was ready to learn any new steps. I would sing at the top of my voice and clap and dance.

And take it for granted that I would do the same come the next wedding. Perhaps even mine?

So what do I do now? I still sing, and I still dance. The music plays and I move my scooter in time with the music. I twist my scooter around in intricate moves. Around and back and a sharp turn to the right and back again then forward.

'Be careful,' someone calls behind me, grabbing onto my shoulder, stopping me.

'Get out of the way, I'm dancing,' I want to shout, gesturing her away.

I am dancing. And in my life I dance. You may not see it, you may not understand or appreciate it, but I am taking my life and dancing with it.

Sometimes we live in a cacophony of jarring sounds and emotions. We are pulled in different directions and seldom find the time to listen to ourselves. If others don't shout at us, we shout at ourselves. I did not enjoy learning ballet when I was young. I could never be delicate. I never had the grace and lightness and innate sense of rhythm that ballet dancers possess. And I do not dance with balletic grace through my life.

There are stops and starts and I trip over my feet. Through the cacophony, I try to make sense of my life. That is all we can do. Life was never meant to be easy. We might find moments of tranquillity, times when we think we fit the final piece into the jigsaw puzzle. But the next moment the puzzle has changed and we have to start all over again.

I read the book *The Road Less Traveled* by M. Scott Peck when I was first diagnosed. It took me a long time to integrate what he had written. He wrote, 'Once we know that life is difficult – once we truly understand and accept it – then life is no longer difficult. Because once it is accepted, the fact that life is difficult no longer matters.'

That is why multiple sclerosis has become inconsequential to my life. My life is difficult. It is frustrating, annoying and sometimes makes me cry. But I do not struggle and bemoan the reality that my life is not easy. I play my own tune and I make music with what I have.

One of my favourite books when I was a child was *Anne of Green Gables*. I sobbed when Anne's beloved guardian, Matthew, died. Life had been mapped out for her, and was beckoning her. And then came the Bend in the Road. Sometimes we plan our future and cannot imagine how the road may bend taking us to unforeseen destinations. Of course I fear the bend in the road. But I have succeeded in negotiating many bends before and I trust that I will negotiate whatever bends may come. And along my way, *May goodness and kindness pursue me all the days of my life* (Psalms 23:1).

But added to that, I pray that I will always shout with glee, 'Get out of the way, I am dancing.'

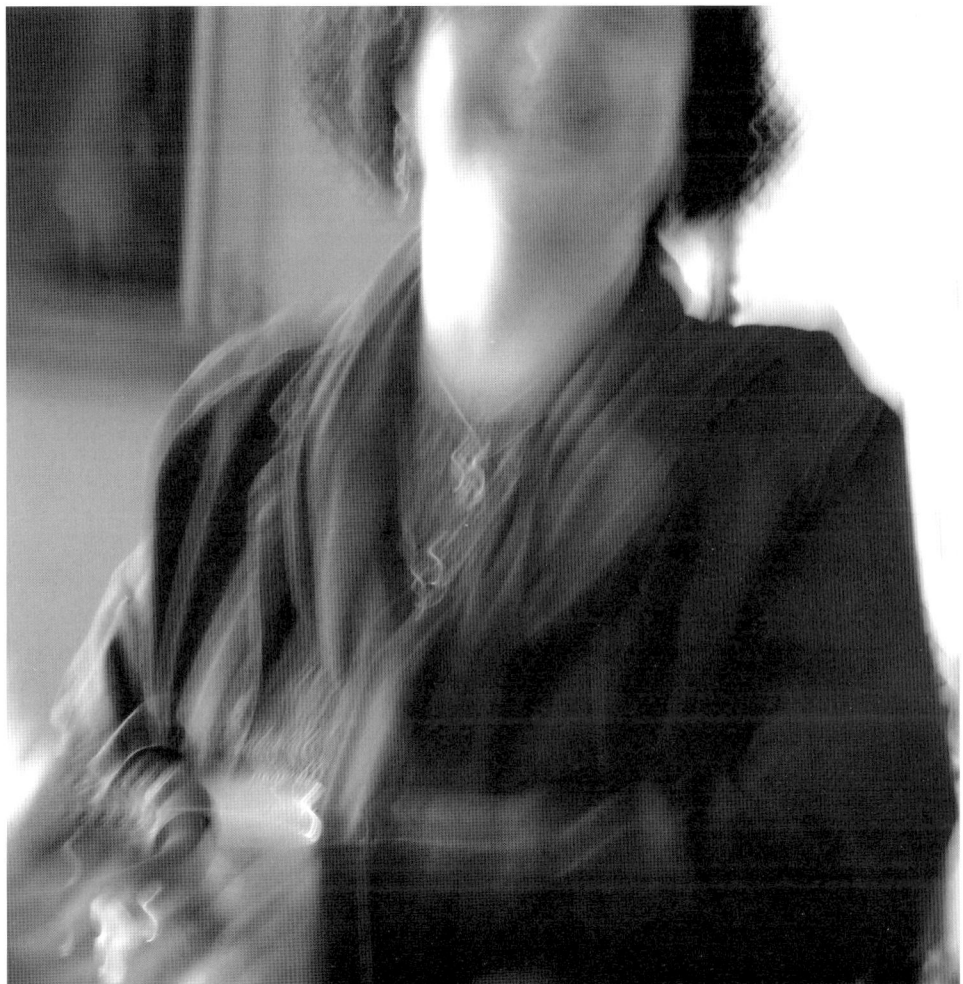

Notes

Notes

Notes

Notes